# His Body, Your Hands

# His Body, Your Hands

## An Illustrated Guide
## to the Art of Erotic Touch

Jeremy Alexander

Charles Beauregard

Also published in French as
**L'Art de caresser un homme: Le guide érotique illustré**

ISBN 978-0-9919001-2-1

## Acknowledgments

We would like to thank the thousands of eager individuals who helped us to produce this guide.

To contact us, please visit our website at

**HisBodyYourHands.com**

# Disclaimer

This guide is intended for educational and entertainment purposes only. The authors, illustrators and editors are not responsible for the use or misuse of any sexual technique or any other suggestion presented in this book, nor for any loss, damage or injury caused by reliance on any information contained in this book. Please use common sense. If you have any health issues or concerns, you should consult a qualified health professional before following any technique or suggestion. Please make sure you follow safer sex practices and consult a qualified health professional if you have any questions. The mention of any sexual aid or device does not constitute an endorsement.

# Table of contents

# YOUR ADVENTURE BEGINS HERE!

*"I wanted to drive him wild with ecstasy, but nothing I did
had much effect…"*

*- A.R.*

You've surely heard the expression *"the way to a man's heart is through his stomach."* Well, it's not true! Most men would prefer an amazing sexual encounter over a good meal that can be easily ordered at a restaurant. To seduce a man, put away your recipe books and read on!

This practical and tasteful guide will help you discover how to enthrall a man with mind-blowing sensual caresses, using just your hands. With a bit of practice, you'll surpass the skills of most people with decades of experience.

In the past, during intimate encounters, you may have asked yourself questions like: *What should I do? How should I begin? Does he like what I'm doing?* It's perfectly normal to wonder about what you're doing and how it feels to him. It's not easy to find good, useful information on how to arouse and intensify male sexual pleasure. We've all heard crude clichés and read glib magazine articles and blogs. Advice on the internet is often unreliable or unrealistic. Friends may be too shy to talk about it, or may know even less than you on the topic.

You could always ask your partner directly, but unfortunately, most men are not very talkative about their intimate feelings. So you may find yourself dealing with a lot of uncertainty, not knowing enough about what he likes, dislikes or has no effect during a sexual encounter. You may be literally guessing in the dark.

The purpose of this book is to help you develop expertise in the art of sexually caressing a man with your hands. You'll understand better than ever how male sex organs function, you'll discover his numerous erogenous zones and broaden your repertory of sexual techniques. With the information in this guide, you can transport your partner to seventh heaven, and his body and soul will exult in the pleasure you produce!

You'll find clearly described techniques that you'll be able to perform with exquisite precision. The trove of information contained in this guide is the result of extensive research, experimentation and interviews with men and women of all legal ages.

We'd like to emphasize an essential point: this guide does not seek to bring a man to orgasm as quickly as possible, but rather, to produce a deep and intensely sensual experience. In our opinion, the path to orgasm is as, if not more, important than the orgasm itself. On the other hand, the skills you'll acquire will allow you to accelerate the process if that is what's desired!

With a bit of practice, you'll master the techniques presented in this book and you'll also discover a large assortment of little tricks that allow you to multiply their effects. You'll soon learn what works best for the man at your fingertips and develop your own signature expertise in the art of erotic touch.

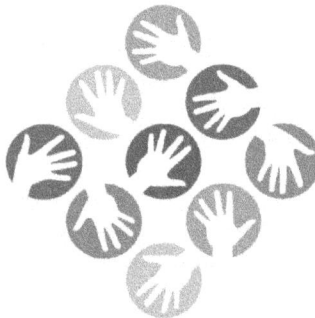

You might be tempted to say: *"That's all very nice...but what about my pleasure in all of this?"* Have no fear! We firmly believe that skilled erotic touching is exciting in and of itself when you see the spectacular results in front of you, and that the time spent perfecting the art of caressing your partner will yield many benefits both inside and outside the bedroom. The same general principles of giving pleasure to your partner are applicable to you, no matter what your gender. In essence, you're showing him by example how to give pleasure. Of course, much depends on how considerate a lover he is, but laying the foundation for reciprocation is an important step. In fact, by serving as an erotic touch role model, we're ready to bet that he'll feel so much gratitude, he'll be quite motivated to satisfy you in return.

As well, we're confident that you'll soon establish more open and direct communication with your partner about what pleases you sexually as well. By welcoming and encouraging regular feedback between yourselves, you'll develop deeper intimacy and trust.

Your intimate encounters will be more enjoyable as you gain confidence and express your erotic creativity. You'll know how to control the tempo and pace yourselves while building up the excitement to a crescendo you've both never before experienced. With your hands, you'll express all the love, desire and respect that you feel for the man who surrenders himself to your expert caresses.

# 10

## good reasons to read this book

1. You want to discover powerfully exciting sexual caresses that few people know about, and become a more skilled and sensual lover.

2. You want to give unforgettably exquisite sensual caresses using only your hands.

3. You've been with the same partner for many years and you want to add fresh excitement to your love life with new erotic techniques and sensations.

4. You'd like to have a sexual encounter with someone but there are certain things you don't want to do (penetrative sex, for example).

5. You might not always have the energy for, or the interest in a complete sexual encounter, but would nonetheless like to indulge him with some intensely satisfying sexual pleasure.

6. You want to be more active, assertive or in control in your sexual encounters (manual caresses are perfect for this!)

7. You love the idea of using his pleasure to toy with him, to excite him or to sexually dominate him.

8. You'd like to have more confidence in the bedroom as you sometimes feel unsure about how to handle a penis.

9. You have more than one sexual partner and you're looking for safer sex techniques.

10. You want to give unprecedented pleasure to a man and make him very happy.

# Legend

An idea or suggestion

Advice on uncircumcised penises

Advice on circumcised penises

Proceed with caution or avoid altogether

A caress or maneuver

Point of information

Reminder

In-depth focus

Message to the whole world

☺☺☺☺☺ Pleasure scale (from 1 to 5 smiles)

**A note on terminology:** We are going to explore several regions of male anatomy, some of which have cumbersome Latin names, or no name at all. To help make these regions easier to identify and remember, we have created custom names. We will use the phrase "...is called..." for official terms and "we call this..." for our own terms.

# THE ANATOMY OF MALE EROGENOUS ZONES

Even though you might be tempted to skip over the first chapters to get to the techniques further in the book, we strongly suggest you read this section first. In the coming pages, we describe some particularly noteworthy aspects of each erogenous zone, and how they can be touched and caressed to significantly augment his sexual pleasure. This information is essential for the mastery of the techniques later on.

Before starting on any journey, you need to know where you're going, and what the terrain will be like. At first glance, you might think you already know about a man's equipment, but please think again! The territory we're going to cover may not be large, but it is quite varied. In fact, many of the erogenous zones that we're going to explore are either underestimated or generally unknown (even by the owner himself!). We're sure you'll agree there are few things more exciting than introducing your partner to a fun part of his anatomy of which he was previously unaware.

To help you get to know the lay of the land, this section will cover:

- The most important male erogenous zones

- Their scientific name or the name that we use in this book to help you remember each

- Their degree of sensitivity and how to stimulate each to maximize his pleasure

- Adjacent regions which can be caressed so as to significantly augment his sexual pleasure

Your future mastery of the techniques presented in this book will depend upon your knowledge of these zones and the type of stimulation that works best on each.

We will start with the most prominent zone and the most well-known: **the penis**.

## What is a Penis?

An odd question! But a worthwhile one.

The answer largely depends on who is asking it, in what context, and who is listening... How would you answer it?

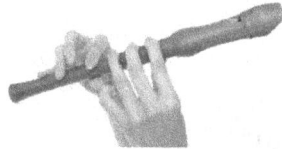

What we've found is that a penis is many things to different people. A penis is:

- An appendage of the male body

- A sexual organ for procreation

- A body part that gives intense pleasure

- An organ for elimination of metabolic waste

- An object of desire

- Man's best friend

- A symbol of fertility

- An object of shame

- An object of worship

- A brutal weapon of aggression

• Ad infinitum....

For the purposes of this book, the penis is a marvelous, organic instrument capable of producing exquisite pleasure, and you are the artist who will master its greatest expression.

Usually hidden from public view, its appearance often provokes a strong reaction. This is anchored in our cultural norms and personal experiences, compounded by the fact that most of us don't often see them "live and in-person". If men did not cover their penises in public life, we would certainly become somewhat more desensitized to the sight of them. While possibly an interesting topic for some, we don't have the time or space here to examine why people react so strongly to a penis, but you might want to observe your own reactions to the sight of a penis, and note if they are positive or negative. Most people have mixed reactions, the greatest determinants being its shape at the moment and the person to whom the penis is attached, quite naturally!

The important thing to remember is that even if you have some negative considerations about the penis *("it's funny-looking"* or *"it smells"),* you can still have loads of good, clean fun with it!

### Did you know...?

*In Greek mythology, Priapus was a god of fertility, and particularly of male genitalia. The son of Aphrodite, he was known for sporting a large, permanent erection.*

*He was paradoxically cursed with impotence, ugliness and foul-mindedness by Hera, another deity and wife of Zeus, while still in his mother's womb.*

*Today, priapism is the medical term for a persistent erection that won't go away. Although this sounds fabulous, this could be a serious condition requiring medical attention.*

# Anatomy of the Penis

No discussion of the functional anatomy of the penis can begin without highlighting the two major varieties of penis that you may encounter. What varieties are these?

- Large and small? No.

- Hard and soft? No.

- Circumcised and uncircumcised? Bingo!

## Circumcision

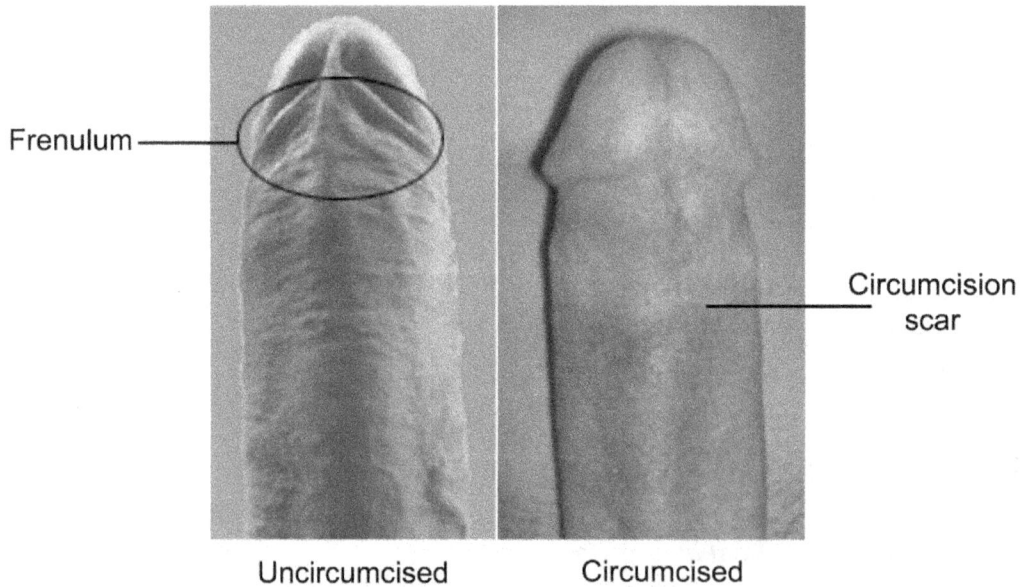

Uncircumcised and circumcised penises

**Circumcision** is the surgical removal of the penile foreskin. It has been practiced for thousands of years by some groups of people in different parts of the world for religious, medical and cultural reasons. There is ongoing debate about circumcision's medical benefits, and whether they outweigh the damage caused by the removal of a significant amount of pleasure-enervated skin. From genital mutilation to the fulfillment of a pact with God, these divergent points of view make this an issue that is both important and controversial. The practice of imposing it on children too young to decide for themselves is, in itself, a serious ethical matter that will no doubt continue to elicit criticism.

Right or wrong, we now have a world full of two kinds of penises. Does it matter to us, in our quest for mastery of male sexual pleasure? Yes, and very much so!

## What's the difference between a circumcised and an uncircumcised penis?

When the **uncircumcised** penis is flaccid, the glans (head) is usually covered by the foreskin, which serves a protective function. The foreskin keeps the glans moist, soft and very sensitive. When the penis is erect, the foreskin slides over the glans and this produces pleasurable sensations. Caressing the uncovered glans of an uncircumcised penis should usually be done gently.

In the **circumcised** penis, the glans is not protected by a foreskin. As a result, it has become relatively desensitized because it is exposed to both friction from clothing and the drying effect of air. Despite its reduced sensitivity (compared to uncircumcised penis), rubbing it can sometimes be painful if your hands are rough or you rub too hard. If possible, try to keep your hands soft or use a lubricant.

**Some other important differences you need to know:**

1. Circumcised and uncircumcised penises function differently during sexual intercourse and other methods of stimulation.

2. On the uncircumcised penis, the foreskin is folded and slides over itself and the head of the penis.

3. Many people commonly refer to a circumcised penis as "cut", and an uncircumcised penis as "uncut" or "intact."

4. Circumcised and uncircumcised penises feel sensations differently and will generally not respond the same way to stimulation techniques. You will need to customize your techniques accordingly. In many of the techniques in this book, we make suggestions for each case.

5. Some uncircumcised men have difficulty retracting the foreskin (pulling it back to expose the head of the penis). You'll need to know if this is the case, as related maneuvers may cause pain or might not be possible.

### ᴼᴼᵔ *How do we know that cut and uncut penises feel differently?*

*Men who've had their foreskin removed as adults have reported this. Many, but not all, note a reduction of pleasure during sexual relations following circumcision. Others experience more pleasure, as previous problems were resolved by the procedure.*

# How can I tell if he's circumcised or not?

Sometimes, it's hard to tell, especially when erect and the foreskin is retracted from the glans. Here's what to look for:

## Uncircumcised

- When erect and the foreskin is retracted, you can see the frenulum, which is a loose or crinkled patch of foreskin that connects to the edge of the glans in front (see picture).
- There is a layer of loose, movable skin covering the glans.

## Circumcised

- You can see the scar line that surrounds the penis below the glans. This scar is a result of the circumcision procedure.

If you're still not sure, don't be shy to ask him. It's not always obvious!

## Circumcision around the world

The prevalence of circumcision varies across the world. Countries with a large proportion of circumcised men include those in the Middle East, Africa and Indonesia. In Europe, South America, Asia, and Russia, circumcision is less common. In North America and Australia, we find both types of men.

### ∞ *Did you know?*

*The 12th century rabbi and physician Moses Maimonides advocated male circumcision for its ability to reduce a man's sexual pleasure and desire (we'll refrain from examining why...). He also opined that once a woman had experienced sexual relations with a lover who was not circumcised, it was very hard for her to give him up!*

## It takes all kinds...

Penises come in different shapes and sizes. Erect penis size varies from less than 7 centimeters (2.5 inches) to over 34 centimeters (13.5 inches). The average penis length is about 15 centimeters (6 inches).

Some penises are straight, some curve up, down or to a side. Some are even corkscrew-shaped. Some are wide in the middle, and taper at the end, others yet are thin, and some have large heads, resembling a mushroom.

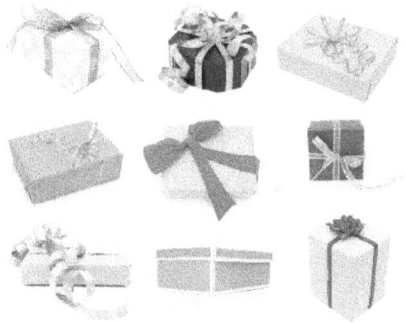

Much has been written and said about penis size and shape. Whether or not it's an issue for you or your partner(s), we offer the following comments:

- All penises are capable of incredible pleasure (unless there is an organic problem).

- Work with the penis you have in front of you, be it large or small, and adapt techniques accordingly.

- Some guys may be shy or embarrassed about the size or shape of their penis, and this may become apparent when it's being looked at or handled. One of your important new skills is to make him feel as comfortable as possible, by treating his penis as wonderfully awesome!

# Name That Body Part!

To help you get better acquainted with the lay of the land, we'll now look at the anatomy of the penis and its surrounding areas. We'll see how these adjacent erogenous zones can be touched and caressed to significantly augment his sexual pleasure.

Your mastery of male erotic pleasure skills will depend on your understanding of these zones and what type of stimulation works best for each. We'll start with the biggest and most famous feature, the penis, but we suggest you also pay particular attention to the other zones, as they make the difference between ordinary and mind-blowing sexual pleasure.

Before we look at our map of masculine paradise, we need to orient ourselves. North, south, east and west don't work well on a 3-D body that can assume an unlimited number of positions. This is especially true of the penis, which can point in many directions.

# The Front of the Penis

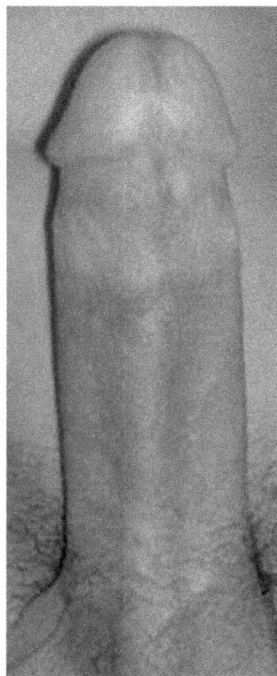

Front of
penis

We'll start at the tip of the erect penis pointing upwards towards his head as you face him. This is officially called the **ventral** side because it's like the belly or underside. In this book, we simply call it the **front** of the penis. The penis above left is uncircumcised, and the one on the right is circumcised.

# The Back of the Penis

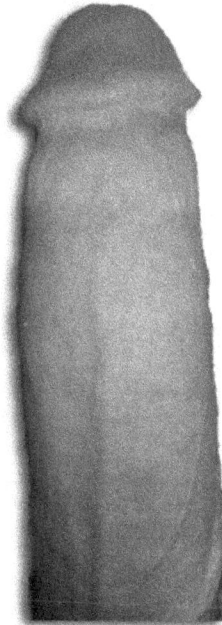

Back of uncircumcised penis          Back of circumcised penis

The opposite side is called the **dorsal** side, or what we call the **back of the penis**. This is the side its owner usually sees when erect. The skin on the back of the penis is generally less sensitive than in front, with the exception of the glans and foreskin.

# The Foreskin

**Pleasure scale (on 5):** ☺☺☺☺☺

Foreskin

It's often the first thing you'll see on an uncircumcised penis, covering the head. It contains tens of thousands of the most pleasure-sensitive nerve endings known to man... and it can be lots of fun to gently play with. As we previously mentioned, it's also what a multitude of men do not have, removed either in infancy or later on in life.

During sexual intercourse or masturbation, the foreskin glides back and forth over the head. This mutual stimulation of head and foreskin produces sublime sensations. The foreskin also allows the penis to be caressed easily without added lubricant.

Its sensitivity to fine touch make it an integral part of sexual stimulation, and there are no end to the ways you can touch it, rub it and make it glide up and down the penis. The frenulum is especially delightful.

Don't despair if he doesn't have a foreskin; the rest of the penis has more than enough pleasure-loving nerve endings to thrill and enthrall!

## *Caresses*

☞ If the foreskin overhangs the penis, you can gently rub the excess foreskin between your fingers, so that the inside of the foreskin slides against itself. This can produce deliriously wonderful feelings.

☞ Gently insert a lubricated finger between the foreskin and the head and caress the head. Make sure you don't have sharp nails!

## The Head of the Penis

**Pleasure scale (on 5):** ☺☺☺

Back of uncircumcised penis                     Back of circumcised penis

Capping the end of the penis shaft is the **glans**, more commonly known as the **head**. Sometimes resembling the cap of a mushroom, it contains a large number of nerve endings, which respond differently than those in the rest of the penis and are more attuned to pressure than to fine touch.

☞ The head loves to be enclosed by the hand, using light to medium pressure.

☞ Adding a partial corkscrew motion adds a nice twist (like you're screwing and unscrewing a light bulb), but limit yourself to quarter-turns or so!

☞ Some circumcised men prefer lubricant when doing this.

In the uncircumcised penis, the foreskin can usually be pulled back to expose the head (although some men find this painful, or are not able to). Be aware that the exposed head on an uncircumcised penis is MUCH more sensitive than the head on a circumcised penis, because the uncircumcised head is used to being protected by the foreskin. So be extra gentle, unless you're told not to be.

When masturbating, most men like to move their foreskin back and forth over the head, uncovering and recovering it, as this is similar to the action that occurs during penetrative intercourse. Use your palm and fingers to grip the foreskin and gently pull it over the head, and then pull it back down. Ask him how far up and how far down he likes it pulled. Some men don't like to have their foreskin retracted.

You can ask him if he likes to have the head rubbed **directly** (without the foreskin between your hand and the head). He may need lubricant for this maneuver. Use less pressure if your hand is rubbing his penis head directly.

Stimulation of the head can be very, very pleasurable, but if you give attention to only the head, its owner may slowly grow frustrated. He may start thrusting his penis so as to get more of it stimulated.

You can have great fun by having him beg you to move down past the head, but make sure you reward him by doing so at least occasionally!

You can achieve greater control by having him lie on his back while you pin down his legs with your thighs, or some variation of this. Use this teasing maneuver with caution (and a bit of mercy)!

# The Meatus

**Pleasure scale (on 5):** ☺☺

Urinary
Meatus

The opening through which the male urinates and ejaculates is called the **urinary meatus**, which is also the end of the **urethra**. For simplicity's sake, you can call it the **pee-hole**.

A clear, viscous fluid called **pre-ejaculate** (or **pre-cum**) is often secreted through this opening when aroused. This natural lubricant can be quite handy, and some men love having a lubricated finger swirl around the opening and adjacent areas. Some men produce significant amounts of pre-cum, and some others produce none at all.

⚠ Be aware that if you are using pre-cum as a lubricant, it dries quickly. If he does not produce enough, the penis can become "tacky" and he will feel an unpleasant friction instead of smooth, gliding pleasure. If this happens, make sure you have extra lubricant standing by!

⚠ In most cases, you should not put anything inside the urethra, unless directed by the owner. If you do go inside, make sure you observe strict rules of hygiene to prevent any infection.

# The Corona

**Pleasure scale (on 5):** ☺☺☺☺

Corona

Notice that the head of the penis flares outward where it joins the shaft. This ridge is called the **corona** (the word derives from the Latin word for crown).

Directly under the corona lies a delightfully pleasurable ring of skin called the **coronal sulcus**. To avoid the awkwardness of having to ask: "Could you please stimulate my coronal sulcus?", we find it more convenient to simply call it the **ridge**.

You can create immense delight when your hand "accidentally" bumps the ridge as you move it up and down the penis.

☞ Using your thumb and index finger as a loose "ring", encircle the penis just under the ridge. Limit your hand to quick, shallow, light up-and-down movements that don't go far down the shaft, essentially just hitting the ridge over and over. Try this with different speeds and pressure to find the combinations that work best.

## The Heart of Pleasure

**Pleasure scale (on 5):** ☺☺☺☺☺

Heart of Pleasure

Front of penis

Moving down the penis, we arrive at the most exquisitely pleasurable region of the male body, second only to the foreskin according to some men. Not surprisingly, we call it the **Heart of Pleasure**. Located on the front (ventral) side of the penis, this heart-shaped sanctum includes a number of smaller zones that we'll look at in more detail.

The skin in the Heart of Pleasure is so sensitive that you usually need to use less pressure than on other zones.

Learning how to stimulate the different regions inside the Heart of Pleasure should be one of your main objectives, so pay extra attention to the following sections. Here you'll find areas that will soon become your favorite buttons on his sexual "remote control"!

# The Teaser

**Pleasure scale (on 5):** ☺☺☺☺☺

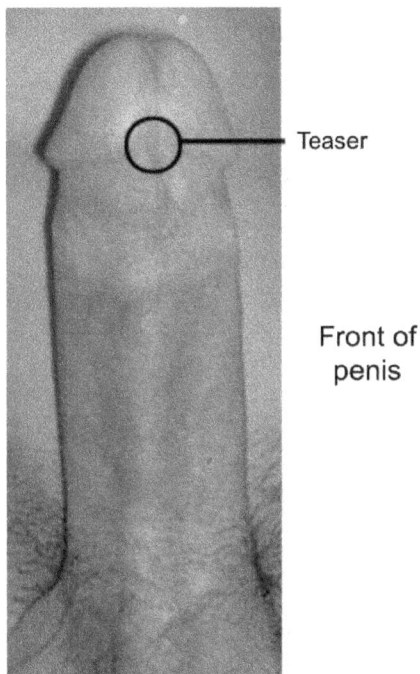

Teaser

Front of
penis

There is an extremely tantalizing spot at the midline of the front of the penis where the head joins the shaft. The anatomy varies between circumcised and uncircumcised males. We call this spot the **Teaser**. This part of the penis is often the first to be stimulated during penetrative sex, and so in addition to feeling really, really good, it has also evolved to send an almost tickling message to his brain that says: *"I want more!"*

🗔 In the uncircumcised penis, (when the foreskin is pulled back), this is a central point where the foreskin attaches to the head. It looks like a loose gathering of skin and is called the *frenulum*.

In the circumcised penis, there is no gathering of skin. However, it is very sensitive and very pleasurable.

In both cases, the Teaser is about the size of a fingernail. Because of its sensitivity, only light to medium pressure should ever be applied here.

A wonderful technique to use on the Teaser is called the **Skating Rink.** It's quite simple and you don't need to sharpen any skates. Using lubrication, slowly circle your finger in small circles on this area. You'll soon see why it's called the Teaser!

# The Sweet Spot

**Pleasure scale (on 5):** ☺☺☺☺☺☺ **(Yes, that's right! It gets 6 out of 5!)**

Sweet Spot

Front of penis

Towards the lower end of the Heart of Pleasure lies the ultimate, most amazingly pleasurable cluster of nerve cells in the male universe, called the **Sweet Spot**. Fortunately, both circumcised and uncircumcised men lay claim to this hallowed ground.

In the uncircumcised penis, the Heart of Pleasure and the Sweet Spot are part of the frenulum. They are alternately covered and uncovered by the back and forth glide of the foreskin. The internal foreskin moves against these zones and this hidden movement of foreskin against penis generates blissful pleasure!

In the circumcised penis, the Heart of Pleasure and the Sweet Spot are always exposed. You can see the scar line (from the circumcision) that circles around the shaft. The scar line marks the end of the super-sensitive and ultra-pleasurable skin.

You can greatly enhance the feel-good response of the Sweet Spot by gently pulling down the skin of the penis at the base of the shaft (towards the testicles). Then gently touch or rub the Sweet Spot. This maneuver, like most of the techniques in this book, works only when the penis is erect.

The Sweet Spot, being so sensitive, can become temporarily desensitized if over-stimulated. This happens in both the circumcised and uncircumcised penis if the foreskin is retracted...too much of a good thing!

Another praiseworthy caress consists of touching a very small part (about the size of a cotton swab stick end) of the Sweet Spot, and then touch another and another, avoiding previously touched areas. This allows continuous pleasure, as it allows nerve endings to rest and "re-charge their pleasure batteries".

*Before going any further, we need to talk about nerve endings and how to best manage their sensitivity...*

# Nerve Endings and Desensitization

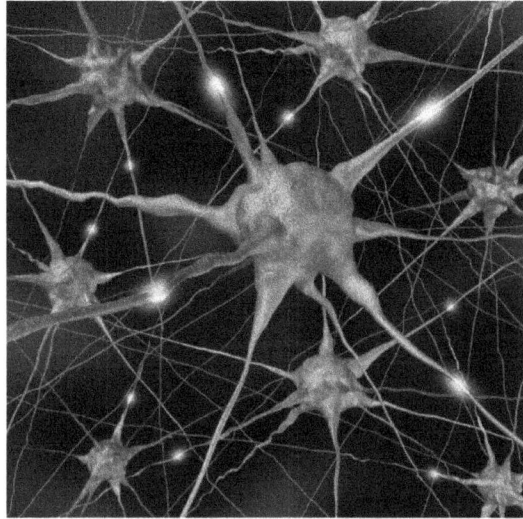

Each time your skin is touched, the affected nerve endings send signals through your nervous system to your brain. If the stimulation is sustained, there is a mechanism in place that causes the nerve response to diminish. For example, when you get dressed in the morning, you are very much aware of the feeling of your clothes on your body, but a few minutes later, you're no longer aware of where your clothes are touching your skin.

It makes sense that if your skin hasn't been touched in a while, you'll feel it more intensely than if it was being touched constantly. This is one of the most important points to remember in the art of erotic touch!

When giving erotic caresses, you want to prevent nerve endings from getting accustomed to stimulation. You can avoid this by alternating the areas you are touching, by pausing briefly between strokes, or by varying the way you touch, changing speed, rhythm or pressure.

# The Ski Runs

**Pleasure scale (on 5):** ☺☺☺☺☺

There are two short strips skin that, when properly stimulated, can make him shudder with delight. They run along both sides of the midline on the front of the penis, on either side of the Heart of Pleasure. We call them **Ski Runs**, because he'll love it when you glide down with your finger. Since they are so close to the Sweet Spot, but slightly away from it, they can enjoy a little more protracted manual stimulation before losing sensitivity. Don't forget: pausing allows the nerves to recover and re-sensitize.

Ski Runs

Front of penis

☞ These parallel stretches of skin enjoy being tickled, lightly brushed, or glided over by a finger while your other hand firmly grips the lower part of the penis shaft (between the base and the Sweet Spot) and slowly strokes it up and down, pulling the loose skin back and forth along the penis. It isn't necessary to stimulate both runs at the same time, and you can alternate between each to make it more interesting.

☞ Stimulating the Ski Runs in a measured and prolonged manner can lead to a very intense sexual build up, and even to a very intense orgasm!

⚠️ **A warning about the circumcised penis (and the uncircumcised penis when the foreskin is retracted):**

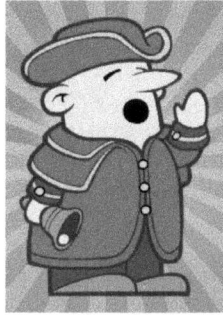

As we've already mentioned, the nerve endings on the penis, and particularly in the most sensitive zones we've just covered, may experience a degree of desensitization resulting from continuous stimulation.

What can you do?

☞ Avoid rubbing these areas continuously or too long or too firmly. Instead, touch them lightly, and pause between caresses.

☞ Alternate by touching other areas to give the nerves in each zone the time to "recharge their pleasure batteries".

💡 Knowing how and when to pause your caresses will dramatically increase his level of sexual excitement!

☝️ Timing is as important to sexual stimulation as it is to stand-up comedy!

# The Shaft

**Pleasure scale (on 5):** ☺☺☺

The **shaft** of the penis, which for our purposes does not include the head or the sensitive area just below it, has relatively fewer nerve endings than the other zones we've explored so far. Moving along the shaft, and heading towards the base, the skin becomes less sensitive to touch, relatively speaking. This presents one big advantage: it's the ideal place you can grip the penis while performing your magic. Here, the penis responds well to a little more pressure.

## *Caresses*

☞ Squeezing the penis. Not too hard! Most penises usually prefer to be squeezed side to side, rather than top to bottom. All around pressure is pleasurable too!

☞ When facing the erect penis pointing upwards, gently grip the lower part of the shaft, just below the Sweet Spot. This allows you to treat the top half of the penis with a multitude of caresses.

For the uncircumcised penis:

☞ With your hand, slowly glide the foreskin over the head of his erection. Stop, then bring it back where you started from, and even a little lower.

Some variation is needed for the circumcised penis:

☞ Grip the lower half of the erect penis with one hand. Slowly move your hand, as well as the skin that it's holding, up towards the head. Once you reach the limit of the skin's elasticity, stop, and bring the skin back to where you started, and even a little lower.

☞ Slide your hand along the shaft of the penis (the skin itself should not move much) towards the top of the head, and then slide it back down. Repeat often. Your partner may prefer this caress to be done with a lubricant. You can do it without, but use a light touch, which will reduce the friction.

# The Base of the Penis

**Pleasure scale (on 5):** ☺☺

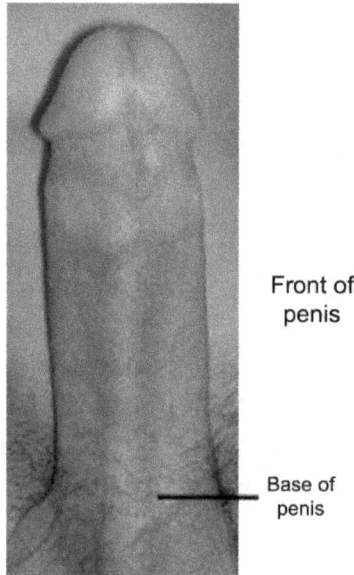

Front of
penis

Base of
penis

Like most of the shaft, the base has fewer fine-touch nerve endings than the head and foreskin. Gripping the base of the penis all around will feel good. Applying gentle pressure underneath and on the sides gives enjoyable results, but front to back pressure (squeezing) can often be unpleasant.

## All done?

We've now reached the point where the penis attaches to the rest of his body. You may think you now have all the knowledge you need to bring your partner to the heights of ecstasy. Not quite yet! There's lots more to discover.

The truth is you've only seen half the attractions. So buckle your seatbelt, take a deep breath and let's keep exploring! Stimulating the areas you're about to see next will really blow his mind!

# The Pubis

**Pleasure scale (on 5):** ☺☺

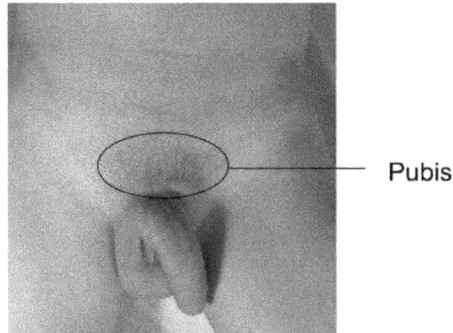

Pubis

In men, the **pubis** is an erogenous zone that is too often neglected. To explore this area, place your hand underneath his navel. Slide your hand down towards the base of the penis. Moving your hand around that area, you should be able to feel a hard, boney surface (the pubic bone) and then a cavity below, just above where the penis is attached to the body. Applying gentle pressure to this and the surrounding area can enhance and augment the pleasurable effects when caressing his penis.

## *Caresses*

This zone responds well to:

☞ Circular motion using the front of your hand, as well as side-to-side and up-and-down, using light to medium pressure.

☞ The light pressure of a kiss, especially when your mouth touches the point where the penis is attached to the body.

If you stimulate the pubis when he is erect and close to orgasm, there is a good chance that he'll ejaculate.

# The Scrotum and Testicles

**Pleasure scale (on 5):** ☺☺☺

Testicles

Scrotum

The **scrotum** is a sack at the base of the penis that contains the **testicles**. Without going into reproductive physiology, here are some important things to remember about these organs:

☞ The testicles are extraordinarily sensitive to pressure and will experience pain beyond a certain point. For this reason, getting kicked in the groin can be an excruciating experience. However, the skin of the scrotum itself is not very sensitive to pain. Be careful when manipulating this area that you don't squeeze the testicles too hard.

☞ The skin of the scrotum is very elastic. When warm, it loosens and stretches, and the balls hang low. When cold, or when ejaculation is near, the scrotum contracts and brings the balls close to the body.

Contracted scrotum

☞ The scrotum has many sensitive touch receptors. Touching, stroking and rubbing the scrotum while stimulating the penis can produce intense pleasure.

☞ Some men trim or shave the hair on their scrotum. This changes the sensation, enhancing it for some. You can suggest to your partner that he shave his balls at least once to experience what it's like. Or better still, you can offer to carefully shave them for him (if you know how to shave) for an unforgettable experience!

# The Perineum and the Inner Creases of the Thighs

**Pleasure scale (on 5):** ☺☺☺

If ever there was an overlooked heavenly oasis on Earth, it's the **perineum**! This is the stretch of skin that runs between the scrotum and the anus. It is a particularly erogenous zone for many men. It's often overlooked and many men have no idea of its potential for enjoyment. Imagine the thrill (and irony) of being the one who introduces it to him!

By itself, it doesn't appear to have any special features, but when the penis is erect and being stimulated, this area responds spectacularly to being touched, caressed or licked. Why, you ask? Honestly, we don't know. But we do know that applying the right techniques at the right time can send your man to Cloud Nine!

There is a central line that runs along the perineum called the **raphe**. It can be felt, and may be seen if there is not too much hair. Adjacent to the perineum are the **creases of the inner thigh**, delightfully sensitive patches of erogenous skin.

The raphe is more easily seen when the scrotum is contracted.

# The Hidden Penis

**Pleasure scale (on 5):** ☺☺☺

*"Appearances can be deceiving."*

*-Aesop (620-560 BCE)*

Suppose you woke up one morning to find your man's penis was 50% longer than you previously thought. What would you say?

 a) I'm still dreaming, don't wake me up!
 b) It's a nightmare!
 c) Stop playing with my head!
 d) Which man are you talking about?
 e) None of the above.

Well, the correct answer is (e) and to that we add: "Good morning!" As you can see from the following diagram, the penis we're all familiar with is only the external, visible portion of a much longer organ. This **hidden penis** is rooted deep in the groin, its tissues extending far back almost to the anus. Significantly, it buttresses the prostate above it.

When the penis is erect, the root of the penis becomes enlarged and stiff as well, and presses against the prostate, stimulating its pressure-sensitive nerve endings. This pleasure, felt deep inside, not only adds to the thrilling sensations, but is an important part of the cascade of neuromuscular reactions that triggers orgasm and ejaculation. On most men, you can feel the hidden penis by placing your hand along the perineum when he is aroused. The area will feel firmer and larger than when he is not.

## What does this mean, from a practical point of view?

- *For one thing, every man's penis is much longer than it appears.*

- *Secondly, you have a lot more real estate to work with!*

## Caresses

☞ You can significantly increase his pleasure by delicately massaging his hidden penis with your fingertips. Start just behind the scrotum and keep going, bit by bit, along the length of the perineum until the anus. You can make small circles, or apply light pressure, or gently roll the loose skin between two fingers. When using this caress at the beginning of a session, go slow. If you're further along, go more quickly. Be careful not to squeeze too hard!

💡 Greater pressure can be applied in the perianal region (the portion of the perineum closer to the anus). In the front half of the perineum, the same pressure can cause discomfort.

☞ Caress or rub the raphe (the central line that runs along the perineum) with one, two or three fingers.

☞ The area where the perineum meets the scrotum contains a great number of fine-touch sensitive nerve endings. When a man is very excited, lightly touching this spot with a finger or two can trigger an orgasm.

☞ Caress the internal creases of the thighs with one, two or three fingers. You can also caress them with your palm, the front or back of your hand, while maximizing the amount of contact between your hand and his perineum. Doing both thighs at once can be quite delightful!

These zones are targeted in many of the techniques described later in this book. Always remember that, for maximum effect, caresses of the perineum should be done when the penis is erect and being stimulated.

We suggest you experiment with caressing the perineum and asking your partner to share about his sensations so you can determine his preferences.

⚠ In some men, the perineum can be ticklish. This can be exacerbated by fatigue or stress. If he can't tolerate your caressing this area, use firmer pressure, or try it another time when he is more relaxed.

## The Anus and the Anal Erozone

We now arrive at a part of the anatomy that, for many, is taboo: the **anus**. We understand that you may not be comfortable with the idea of caressing this part of your partner. Certainly, everyone is entitled to their point of view. Some heterosexual men do not want their anus touched, even by a woman, because they associate anal pleasure with homosexuality. Ironically, there are many gay men who are not at all interested in anal sex.

To give fair consideration to all the intense pleasure it has to offer, it's worth exploring this erogenous zone with your partner. You can always come back to play in the other zones if either of you is uncomfortable. But in the name of knowledge, enlightenment and pure hedonistic ecstasy, everyone should at least consider the powerfully exciting sensations that are possible here.

The male anus has two attributes that make it a powerful erogenous zone:

1. A large number of exquisitely sensitive nerve endings line the anus. Some of these nerves extend outside the anus, into the perianal area, which we call the **Anal Erozone**.

2. The anus gives access to an organ that is crucial to sexual pleasure: the **prostate**.

## Exploring the Anal Erozone

**Pleasure scale (on 5):** ☺☺☺

Anal Erozone

Caressing the external Anal Erozone with your fingers or the back or palm of your hand can produce wonderful sensations. The skin immediately surrounding the anus is richly enervated, and this increases as one approaches the anus. Some men love this kind of stimulation. It may make others tense, either because they find it distracting, or they may have negative considerations about this area, related either to hygiene or fear of homosexual connotations about enjoying these sensations.

### *Caresses*

☞ Gentle, slow caresses are very pleasurable. You will need to get feedback from him for stronger movements.

☞ Putting a bit of lubricant on a finger and gently swirling it around the entrance of the anus, without penetration, can dramatically escalate pleasure while manipulating the penis.

Caressing this zone without an erection present, or without stimulating the penis at the same time, may not produce any of these wonderful sensations.

You can explore the area around your own anus with your finger to get an idea of what it feels like for your partner. However, if you are a woman, it will not be exactly the same, as you don't have a prostate.

# The Anus: A Shrinking Violet

**Pleasure scale (on 5):** ☺☺☺☺

The anus on most men is like a shrinking violet: it's shy, sensitive and needs to be slowly encouraged to relax.

There is not one but two sphincter muscles that surround the anal canal. The external sphincter is under voluntary control, and it's what you contract when you want to prevent defecation. The internal sphincter is under the control of the autonomic (involuntary) nervous system, and we have very little control over it. Even though you cannot contract and relax your internal sphincter at will, you can learn to release it using basic relaxation exercises.

## Exploring the Anus

You need to be patient with this area, and if you want your partner to experience the numerous pleasures associated with it, you'll need to go slowly and gently.

⚠️ **Be careful with long or sharp fingernails!** If you want to keep your fingernails long, you'll need to find another object to use instead. There are many dildos and prostate massagers available at sex shops and online which are carefully designed for this purpose. In this case, it's always best to start with something small, around the width of a finger. Avoid using household objects that may tear the delicate lining, or might get lost inside!

☞ Caress the external anal region and slowly edge your way towards the anus. Take your time so that he can get used to the presence of your finger in this intimate area and to allow the sphincters to relax.

☞ Next, gently slide your lubricated finger into his anus to at most one or two centimeters (a half inch or less). After a second or two, slowly withdraw your finger. You'll need to pay attention to his reactions, as his sphincters may be tense, and if so, will not allow your finger to penetrate.

☞ If he doesn't have any negative reaction, you can slowly and gently penetrate his anus again. Remember: There is no rush!

☞ Observe all of his reactions: his respiration, facial expressions and body language. If he's tense, it may be (but not necessarily) because you went too quickly. Stop, refocus your caresses on another zone, and then try again a few minutes later. If you're not sure, you can always ask.

☞ You don't have to insert your finger completely for him to have pleasurable sensations. Some men prefer that the finger stays just outside the anus. Others prefer that the finger penetrates only to the first joint.

☞ Some men like a bit of finger movements inside: this can vary from occasional finger twitch to a gentle finger massage to full in-and-out motion. Others prefer simply the sensation of a finger there, without any movement at all, while their penis is being manipulated.

☞ After a certain amount of time, even a motionless finger can cause some discomfort. To avoid this, withdraw your finger, give it a rest, and come back later for another visit.

⚠ If you proceed too rapidly (when he is not ready, without using enough lubricant, or you have sharp nails), this may trigger a reflexive clampdown, and you may never get another invitation again!

💡 Nothing could be more enlightening than trying this on yourself to gain an idea of what it feels like!

💡 For added safety, you can use a finger cot, which is like a small latex condom for your finger. You can find these at most pharmacies.


If your partner finds penetration painful, ask him to push out his anus as if he was trying to defecate. This helps the internal sphincter to relax, and should stop the pain.

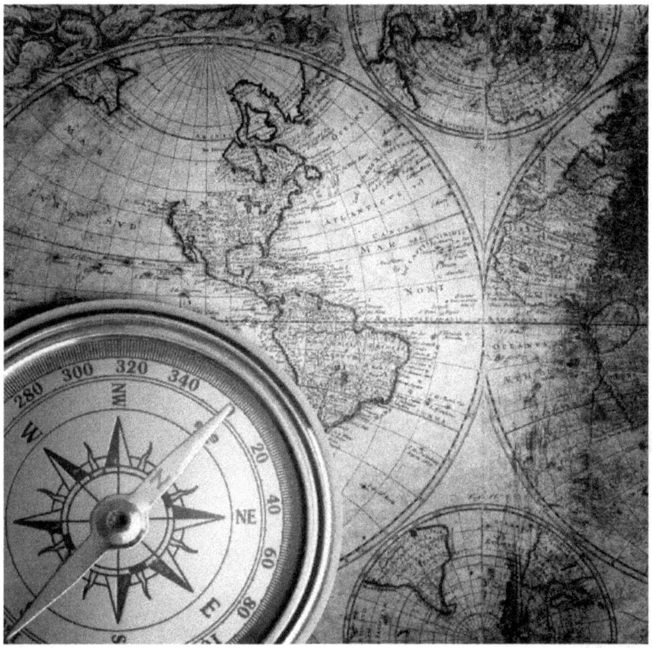
280
300
320
340
NW
W
NE
20
40
60
80
E

## Safety Tips

If you and your partner wish to expand your erotic horizons to include anal pleasures, by using either a finger or some other non-hazardous object, always take basic safety precautions:

☝ It's always a good idea to wash the anus with soap and water before touching the area. Additionally, if you plan to insert your finger into the anus, you can ask your partner to cleanse his rectum (anal canal) with a warm-water rectal douche. You can easily find enema bulbs online or at your local pharmacy. While not absolutely necessary, this cleansing may be appreciated by some.

☝ Make sure your hands and all objects used are clean.

☝ Never use anything with sharp or rough edges. The mucous membrane is only one cell thick, and can easily be torn.

☝ Always use plenty of lubricant when penetrating the anus.

Never force anything, in any direction.

Never insert anything that can be 'lost'. Make sure that the object has a part that is too wide to enter. We recommend using fingers or reasonably size sex toys designed for this purpose, and to avoid household objects and vegetables.

The anus may contain bacteria such E. Coli, hepatitis, or parasitic organisms. If you don't know the health status of your partner, please be extra prudent.

If you don't want to touch the anus, you can still produce pleasurable sensations by stimulating the prostate using indirect means. We will explore this possibility in the next section.

# The Prostate

**Pleasure scale (on 5):** ☺☺☺☺☺

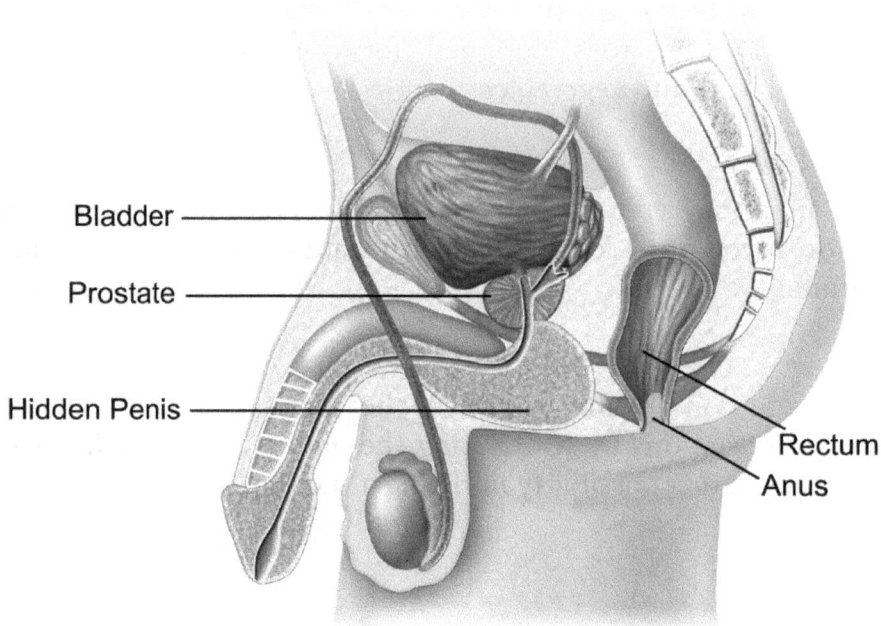

One of the best kept secrets of male sexuality is the important role of the prostate in sexual sensations and orgasm.

Situated just above the root of the penis, the prostate is, without question, the second most important sexual organ in men. It is considered by some to be the equivalent of the "G-spot" in women.

You'll note in the above diagram that the prostate is situated very close to the front wall of the rectum. In fact, if you insert your middle finger into the rectum of your partner when he is facing you, and if your finger is long enough, you should be able to feel the prostate. It feels like a firm, round mass approximately the size of a large cherry tomato on the other side of the rectal wall.

The prostate has too many important functions to cover here. We'll mention only those that can be useful:

☝ During sexual arousal, the prostate senses gentle pressure as pleasure (but too much pressure can be uncomfortable or painful).

☝ Much of its pleasurable sensations are caused by indirect pressure transmitted by adjacent tissues.

☝ The pleasurable sensations mediated by the prostate are different from, but can be just as intense, as the sensations experienced by the penis.

☝ During ejaculation, the prostate contracts and its contractions are an important part of the orgasm.

☝ Orgasms that occur when the prostate is being stimulated are usually more intense and powerful.

Here are some ways to stimulate the prostate:

**Indirectly**:

☞ Pressure from the root of the penis (the hidden penis).

☞ Manipulating (changing the angle of) the erect penis upwards, downwards, or from side to side.

☞ Contractions of the lower pelvic muscles can squeeze the prostate. **Kegel** exercises can be performed to strengthen these muscles and maintain their muscle tone. These exercises involve alternatively clenching and releasing the pubococcygeus (PC) muscle. This is the muscle that activates when you try to stop the flow of urine when urinating. The muscle exists in both men and women. Another way to identify your PC muscle is to insert a lubricated finger in your anus and use the anus to grip the finger.

☞ Gentle upward pressure applied in the perianal zone (the perineum close to the anus) using your fingers or your hand.

**Directly**:

☞ Direct prostate massage using a finger inserted in the rectum.

☞ Prostate massage using a dildo. One can find a wide variety of sexual objects online that can be used to massage the prostate.

☞ Anal intercourse between men stimulates the prostate directly.

The advantage of using a finger is that it can feel the prostate become firmer just prior to orgasm and this will permit you to be more precise and timely in your caresses.

⚠ Prostate massage, when done with a finger or sex aid, should always be done gently. Too much pressure can be uncomfortable or painful. The prostate is normally protected from trauma by its location deep inside the pelvis, so please be prudent when handling it!

## Caresses

☞ Use your middle finger because it's the longest and will allow you to reach the prostate. It's possible that it might not be long enough. If this is the case, you can try using a dildo or prostate massage aid.

☞ Move your finger gently around the contours of the prostate going from left to right or from top to bottom.

☞ Ask your partner for feedback about how much pressure to use.

☞ Lightly tap the prostate with your finger.

☞ Some men like having a second finger inserted as well. Some others like even more!

☞ You can press the side of your whole hand against the outside of the anus. This gentle pressure also produces enjoyable sensations.

☝ If your finger is in contact with his prostate when he ejaculates, you will feel contractions of the prostate. After ejaculation, remove your finger very slowly. Quick removal can be uncomfortable!

Don't be alarmed if he makes noises that you've never heard before. The pleasure can be deep and powerful!

**Tip**: "Sit on my...knee!"

A useful, but unthreatening way for him to identify the pleasurable prostate effect is to masturbate him (or have him masturbate himself) in a standing position with you sitting in a chair in front of him. Ask him to assess how much pleasure he is feeling on a scale from 1 to 10.

Next, ask him to sit on your knee still facing you, with one leg on either side of your leg, while continuing the exact same stimulation as when standing. Ask him to re-assess his pleasure. Any increase in delight is due to the indirect pressure of your knee on his prostate.

For more details, please see the technique **Sit on my knee** in the Techniques section.

You now have a powerful new key to his sexual ecstasy!

# The Leverage Point

**Pleasure scale (on 5):** ☺☺☺☺

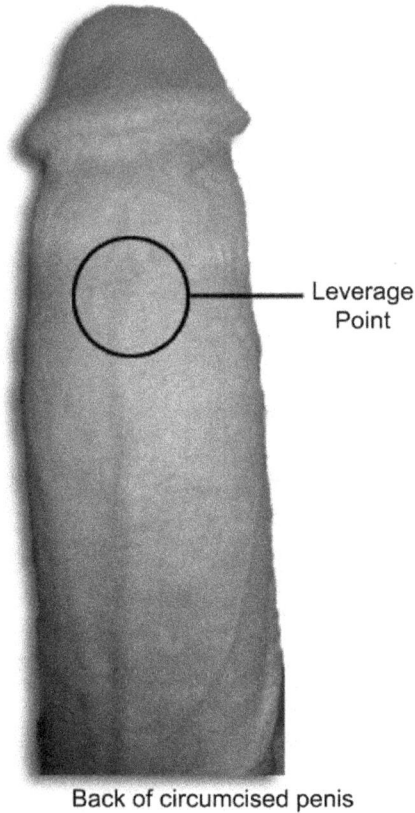

Leverage
Point

Back of circumcised penis

The zone that we called the **Leverage Point** is an area the size of an American quarter, located on the back of the penis, about one-third of the way down the shaft. In the circumcised penis, it is at the level of the scar line. This is an unusual zone because it's not so much the sensitivity of the skin that gives pleasure, but the effect of gently pressing on the penis at this point that causes sexual pleasure to be felt all over the penis and within the pelvis too!

How is this possible?

When the penis is erect, its root (the part that is inside the body) lies very close to the prostate. By gently rubbing the leverage point and pushing the penis slightly down towards his feet, you are stimulating the entire organ from top to bottom, and placing highly enjoyable indirect pressure on the prostate. These actions excite nerve endings located deep inside the groin, which interpret these signals as those associated with sexual intercourse.

It's simple and effective. It's the pleasure lever!

**Leverage his pleasure!** You can activate the Leverage Point in a few ways:

☞ Using a finger or hand, press down on the erect penis by touching only the Leverage Point, pushing his penis towards his feet.

⚠ Careful: There is a limit to how far down you can press, beyond which you'll produce discomfort or pain. You'll learn from his reaction, or by asking him, exactly where is his limit.

☞ You could also move the skin gently around in a small circle using your finger. You can do this when the penis is standing freely, or for extra oomph, try it when the front of his penis is pressed against your other hand, his leg, or something else. You'll be amazed at how good he feels with this simple maneuver!

Remember – this leverage effect only works when the penis is hard. A semi-hard penis will probably not feel much effect from this maneuver.

Don't be surprised if he closes his eyes and moans. He's not suffering – he's in paradise!

# The Hidden Penis Revisited

Earlier, we explored the hidden penis and its proximity to the prostate. Let's explore how you can stimulate the prostate by manipulating the hidden penis in a number of ways.

### 1. The Pressure Method:

☞ With your hand, or other soft object, gently press up against the back half of the perineum (close to the anus). This puts pleasurable pressure on the prostate.

### 2. The Leverage Method:

The best way to understand this maneuver is to picture a see-saw. A see-saw is essentially a long lever, balanced upon a fulcrum at its midpoint. When there is more weight on one side, or the center of gravity shifts further out to one side than the other (by leaning back), that side drops down and the other side rises.

The penis can be seen as a see-saw. But we're talking about the whole penis, including its hidden root. The mid-point of the penis is approximately where it joins the body. This means that the visible, external penis is one half of the see-saw, and the hidden penis is the other half.

☞ Visualize an erect penis on a standing man. If you pull the penis gently DOWN, you should be able to imagine the other, hidden end of it going UP. So what, you ask? When it goes up, it presses against the prostate and produces deep pleasure. But there's a limit... You'll need to learn how much pressure he likes, and what is the maximum angle before the pleasure turns to discomfort.

☞ Other variations of this method include: gently pulling the erect penis from side to side, diagonally and directions in between. Your tactic here is to change the angle of the erection relative to the body. You can also gently pull it out and away from the body.

☝ **Tip:** A good place to press on is the Leverage Point (explored in the previous section).

## The Axis of Pleasure

**Pleasure scale (on 5): Varies from** ☺ **to** ☺☺☺☺

If you think, as we do, that there's too much pain, suffering and evil in the world, then you'll be happy to know that every man has his own built-in antidote. It's called the Axis of Pleasure!

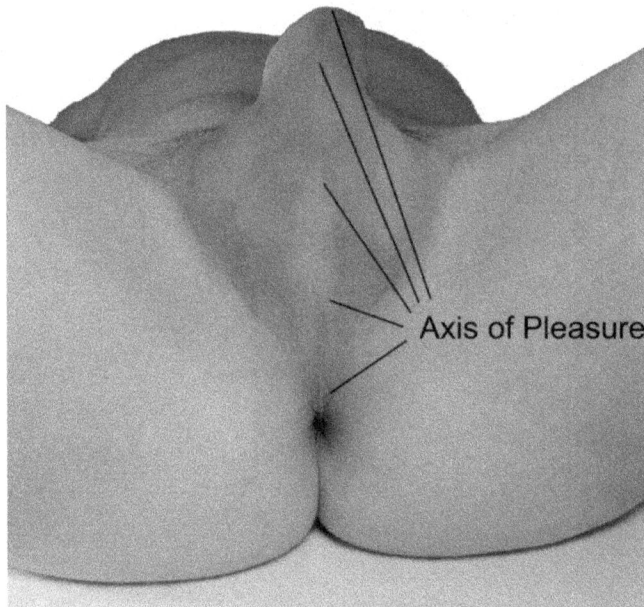

Axis of Pleasure

Now that you have an overall view of the male erogenous zones in the genital area, the **Axis of Pleasure** will help you to:

- Remember these zones more easily

- Understand how these zones are interrelated

The Axis of Pleasure follows a central line of sometimes ridged, sometimes bumpy, sometimes darker flesh that has the appearance of a seam where the two lateral halves of the body join at the groin, otherwise generally known as the **raphe**. Though perhaps not as visually spectacular as the Great Wall of China, this line still spans a lot of sexual geography.

The Axis extends from the tip of the penis, down along its front underside, through the mid-line of the scrotum and perineum, into the anus and ending inside at the highest point on the prostate.

What's important to know about this line is its nerve endings are more pleasurable and sensitive than the surrounding skin. Generally speaking, caresses along most points of the Axis can be spectacularly exquisite when the penis is hard and being stimulated by hand, mouth or penetration.

## Take a tour along the Axis of Pleasure!

👆 The first section of the Axis, starting from the tip of the penis, runs through the most sexually sensitive zones of skin in the male: the Teaser, the Heart of Pleasure and the Sweet Spot.

👆 As we head down the mid-shaft, the Axis seems to disappear, but rematerializes at the scrotum, where it continues down and around. Caresses along the scrotal raphe can be entrancing!

👆 As you move from outlying areas towards the Axis, the intensity of pleasure increases.

👆 In many men, the Axis along the perineum is particularly sensitive. It responds well to light to medium stroking.

The point at which the Axis meets the anus often loves to have a lubricated finger gently massage it.

The significance of the Axis of Pleasure cannot be overstated. Like a sexual fault line, this is where orgasmic earthquakes can be triggered!

## The Inner Thighs

**Pleasure scale (on 5):** ☺☺☺

As we all know, the inner thighs can be very sensitive to touch. They are reflexively perceived by most people as an extremely intimate area, and form an often overlooked erogenous zone that you can use to heighten a man's pleasure.

Since some parts of the inner thigh can be ticklish, some men may prefer a firm, steady hand, instead of a light, grazing touch. You'll need to discover for yourself what your partner prefers.

Stimulation of the inner thighs can be very erotic at the beginning of a session, before you've even touched the penis.

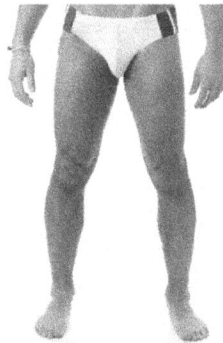

### *Caresses*

☞ Starting halfway down the thigh, slowly stroke your hand upwards along the inner thigh. Your partner will enjoy the anticipation of your hand slowly moving towards his genitals, hoping that it will eventually touch them. It may be fun to tease him with this for a while, but don't make him squirm for too long!

☞ Draw small or large circles around the inside leg with the palm of your hand, occasionally brushing against the perineum and the anus.

☞ While touching the penis, rub an inner thigh with your other hand in circular, or up-and down motions. You can also bring your hand up to the inner crease of the thigh and perineum.

☞ The feeling of a hand firmly gripping the inside thigh is pleasurable for many men.

☞ You can use both hands to apply light-to-medium pressure on his inner thighs, as if you were trying to spread his legs. Some men find this very pleasurable, and the increased exposure of his genitals can add to his feelings of excitation.

# The Buttocks

**Pleasure scale (on 5):** ☺☺☺

The buttocks are one of the most scrutinized body parts. Both men and women look at them when evaluating the attractiveness of a potential partner. Even though they are tough and can take a spanking, they have areas which are very sensitive to touch and pressure, and these can be used to increase sexual pleasure.

## *Caresses*

☞ The sensitivity of touch receptors increases as you move towards the center of the buttocks, the inner thigh and anus. Cupping the flesh in your hand, stroke or massage the buttock, using circular motion.

☞ Slide your hand along the curves. Allow a finger or two to brush against the Anal Erozone, or the anus itself.

☞ Since the part of the buttock that one sits upon is used to a lot of pressure, the occasional slap on the buttock can be exciting and invigorating for many, and the noise can add a certain frisson.

☞ Squeezing one or both buttocks while stimulating the penis can significantly increase a man's pleasure.

☞ Squeezing a buttock while massaging the Anal Erozone with your other hand can also be very enjoyable.

☞ Spreading the butt cheeks apart as you massage them is a sensation that some men really like.

## Other Erogenous Zones

There are many other erogenous zones, including the chest, nipples, ears, feet, toes and neck, to name a few. We will be discussing some of these in later sections. We urge you to explore the possibilities on your own as every man has his particular erogenous zones and these can vary greatly.

## The Tour is Over!

Yes, we've now come to the end of the anatomy tour. You should now have a good understanding of the diverse male erogenous zones and how to caress them. But before jumping into the various techniques, it's important to learn about the many factors that will affect how your caresses are received and experienced.

# GET READY: Tools and Practical Advice

You now have a good overview of the various male erogenous zones. You may want to start trying out the techniques with your partner right away. However, we strongly suggest you first read the following section, where we explore the many factors that can impact your performance of the techniques.

You'll discover how both pressure and timing affect pleasure, how to adapt your style to the type of partner you have, body positions, the choice of lubricants, the art of using pauses to augment pleasure, as well as how to listen to non-verbal cues. You'll also gain a better understanding of other essential aspects of giving and intensifying sexual pleasure in the male.

Knowing the various elements involved in giving pleasure will allow you to use them in the right way, at the right moment. Sometimes, the simplest touch can produce the most electrifying reaction.

This section is full of useful tools and tips. By taking the time to read it, you can be sure that your partner will come to know he is in the hands of an expert who has mastered a thousand sublime caresses!

# The Male Sexual Response Cycle

Before we go any further, let's quickly look at what happens to a man when he's sexually stimulated. There are four phases in what is known as the Human Sexual Response Cycle. Devised by the famous sex researchers Masters and Johnson, here briefly are the male physiological responses associated with each phase:

## 1. Excitement Phase

The beginning of the sexual response. Heart rate, breathing rate and blood pressure increase. Nipples may become erect. The skin may flush. The anal sphincters may have contractions. The penis becomes partially or fully erect. The scrotum contracts and the testicles move closer to the perineum.

## 2. Plateau Phase

The period of sexual excitement prior to orgasm. The urethral sphincter contracts to prevent urine from mixing with the semen. Muscles in the groin around the penis contract rhythmically. Some pre-ejaculatory fluid may drip from the urethra.

## 3. Orgasmic Phase

The climax. This stage follows the plateau phase and is characterized by waves of intense pleasure, ejaculation of semen, involuntary contractions of muscles surrounding the penis, in the groin, the anal sphincters and sometimes muscles throughout the body, and vocalizations.

## 4. Resolution Phase

Following orgasm, blood pressure, heart rate and respiration normalize. During this period, the penis may be sensitive to touch, and continued stimulation can be unpleasant. Some men, however, can return to sexual activity after a short period of time.

# Essential Tools: Your Two Hands

You have, in your possession, two of the most amazing marvels of evolutionary engineering in the universe. The dexterity of the human hand, with its opposable thumb, has enabled us to develop fine motor skills and create a mind-boggling variety of tools that have propelled us to the moon and back.

The same two hands that can be trained to play the violin and piano, perform brain surgery and build a Swiss watch can also be trained to bring intoxicating pleasure to a man. It's all just a question of knowledge and practice.

## Which parts to use?

- Your fingertips

- The back of your hands, or your palms

- The sides of your hands

• Your fist

• Your wrist

• You can stimulate larger areas using your palm along with the inside wrist, which form a large cup.

Don't forget you can also use other parts of your body, like the tip of your nose, your mouth, tongue, head, elbows, and for some enthusiasts, your feet! There are no limits other than your flexibility.

While caressing your partner, and especially his penis, you'll need to take into account the following elements:

• **pressure**

• **rhythm**, which has two components:

    • speed

    • frequency

• **friction** (rubbing vs. displacing skin)

We'll now look at each of these more closely.

## Pressure: *Squeeze Me!*

**Question:**
How much pressure should I use?

**Answer:**
This depends on **when** you exert the pressure and **where** you're exerting it. Generally, it's preferable to begin a session using a lighter touch, then slowly increase pressure over time, until you want him to reach orgasm. Remember that each body part responds differently to pressure, and you're working inside a continuum where, at one end, a light pressure may have no effect, and at the other end, a heavy pressure can cause discomfort or pain. In between, there is a "Goldilocks" range of pressures that produces pleasure.

Believe it or not, you can sometimes give ten times more pleasure using one-tenth the effort . . . another secret in the art of erotic touch!

To give you a better idea of the levels of pressure to use in your caresses, here is our pressure scale:

0  no pressure
1  holding an egg
2  squeezing a peach to see if it's ripe
3  squeezing an avocado to see if it's ripe
4  squeezing the tube of toothpaste onto the toothbrush
5  closing a zip lock bag

6  opening a car door handle

7  stirring a spoon in a jar of peanut butter

8  applying the brakes in a car

9  holding a jar tightly while opening the lid for the first time

10 holding on to the security bar on a careening rollercoaster

Knowing how much pressure to use, and when, and where, are key skills to master when caressing your partner. With practice and good feedback, you will become quite adept.

# Speed

As with using pressure, it's always a good idea to start slowly, as this gives you the freedom and latitude to speed up later. Normally, in sexual encounters, speed is not constant, and varies according to mood, preference and how long you want the session to last.

# Frequency

Frequency is a function of time. It refers to how many times you perform a particular movement in a given time period. There are no limits to the range of frequencies you can employ, but here's a list of possibilities to give you a better idea:

Once every 10 seconds

Once every 5 seconds

Once every 2 seconds

Once every second

## Rhythm: an Erotic Dance

The relationship between speed and frequency is what we call **rhythm**.

The effect of rhythm on sexual pleasure is powerful and should not be underestimated. Your rhythm should be coherent and follow an improvised or loose pattern. In other words, avoid varying your movements too much to the point of being chaotic or jarring. On the other hand, there should (usually) be a difference between the rhythm at the beginning of your session and at the end. As in dance, rhythm is half learned and half intuitive.

Here are some examples that illustrate variations in rhythm:

☞ Move your hand very **slowly** from the tip of the penis to the base. Then, without pausing, move it very slowly back to the tip. Repeat the same movement without pausing.

☞ Do as above, but pause for a few seconds when your hand is at the tip and at the base of the penis.

In this example, the **speed** is the same but the **frequency** is greater in the first example. Varying the speed of your hand movements and the length of the pauses allows you to create unlimited, diverse rhythms. In dance, you follow the music. Here, you follow your own creative erotic energy and the feedback from your partner. Rhythm is one of the most important principles in building and maintaining erotic momentum.

A good example of this is the musical piece *Bolero* by the composer Ravel (used in the soundtrack of the movie '10'). It starts off slowly, with both the volume and the tempo increasing towards a climactic finale.

## Ah! How sweet it is to do nothing!

Why rush? Take a break. Finally, here's where doing less is more . . . and better. We normally exert lots of effort and determination into activities where we want to excel. You might think that, here as well, touching more would be better, but this is not the case. A pause between two caresses actually makes the second caress more satisfying. When you drink a glass of wine, you don't drink it all in one big gulp. You pause between sips and this makes the experience a lot more enjoyable. It's the same principle with erotic caresses.

It's very important to include pauses during your caresses, particularly on the penis, so that the nerve endings can re-sensitize themselves, as mentioned previously in the section: *Nerve Endings and Desensitization*.

How long is the ideal pause? There is no single answer. Here again, you'll need to rely upon your own experience and the reactions of your partner. The length of the pause will depend upon which stage of sensual play you are at, how excited your partner is, the technique and the rhythm that you've just been using. In general, a pause can last between ½ second and 10 seconds. You should be able to evaluate the effect of the pause by his reaction to the following caress.

When you use the techniques described later in this book, varying the duration and frequency of your pauses will add depth and intensity to his experience of the technique. As well, inserting pauses into your sexual play makes it far more interesting by drawing out moments of anticipation and augmenting his pleasure when he finally receives the caress he is expecting.

Of course, there are times when rapidly jacking a penis like a piston feels really good, particularly towards the end of an erotic session. However, it's only one of a multitude of techniques you'll have at your fingertips.

A fun alternative to a complete pause is to caress another of his erogenous zones during the break and then to come back to the previous zone at the end of the break.

One of the biggest mistakes to avoid is to start masturbating a penis quickly, with lots of pressure. By doing this, you lose the ability to slowly build up pleasure. It's like serving a very sweet, rich dessert at the beginning of a fine gourmet meal. Your guest won't be able to savor the delicate flavors served afterwards.

# The Great Penis Dilemma: *Rubbing* or *Displacing* the Skin?

Most of the techniques used on the penis can be performed by either **rubbing** or **displacing the skin**. There is a subtle but important distinction between the two methods. To help you understand the difference, here is an example of each:

Imagine you have a headache and you are massaging your temples with your fingers such that you are moving the skin around in small circles, as if it were glued to your fingers. This is what we call **displacing the skin**. In this movement, there is no friction between your fingers and the skin of your head.

Imagine now that you are spreading skin cream onto your arm. The skin on your arm does not move around very much, rather, it is your hand that is sliding across the skin of your arm. In this case there is some friction. This is what we call **rubbing**.

Uncircumcised men have lots of very mobile skin and generally prefer having the skin displaced (moved) on their penis. It's the natural movement during vaginal intercourse.

With circumcised men, preferences vary. Some circumcised penises are too sensitive for the rubbing method, which can cause discomfort and skin irritation. For many (but not all), using a lubricant is essential. Always start with a light hand and ask your partner to give you feedback as you increase pressure. Alternatively, you can use the displacement method on a circumcised penis, but bear in mind that the absence of a foreskin leaves you with less skin to move around. Both methods can be exquisitely pleasurable when done well. Monitor the range of motion so that you stay within his comfort zone.

You can also apply these two methods to caressing his other erogenous zones.

⚠ If your hands are dry and rough, it's usually better to avoid rubbing his skin, and to use the displacement method instead.

# What Type of Lover is He?

There are at least five sensory types of lovers: kinesthetic, auditory, visual, olfactory and oral. Simply put, kinesthetic lovers like touching and being touched, auditory lovers are excited by sounds, visual lovers like watching what is going on (and sometimes being watched), olfactory lovers are turned on by odors, and oral lovers get much of their pleasure from using their mouth. Many people are a combination of a few or all of these, but for most of us, one or two types predominate.

Recognizing what kind of lover you're with allows you to adjust your repertoire and radically magnify the excitation effects of your caresses. The same technique can produce a more intense effect if you adapt it to his personality. For example, a predominantly visual lover will experience far more pleasure from a caress when he can see you than if you were in the dark. An auditory lover will enjoy the same caress more if it is accompanied by your amorous sounds or verbalizations. Let's look at each in greater detail.

## The Kinesthetic Lover

The kinesthetic lover likes touching and being touched, finding it profoundly pleasurable. Of all the types, this one will be the most enthralled by the techniques and caresses in this book. Some like light, sensual caresses, others prefer more robust handling, and there are some who like to be tickled or to feel pain.

Some helpful tips to intensify his pleasure:

👆 Start with a massage.

👆 Use a great variety of the techniques presented in this book.

👆 Caress his body everywhere, even zones which are not generally considered erogenous.

👆 He may surprise you by rapidly integrating the principles and techniques you've learned in this book, without reading it, when he caresses you.

## The Auditory Lover

The auditory lover is not only excited by caresses, but also by the sounds he hears and makes.

When caressing him:

👆 Emit moans or purrs.

👆 Talk to him while caressing him. Learn what kinds of talk excites him: romantic, erotic, role-play, naughty or other. This should be discussed beforehand so that both of you are comfortable and enjoy the experience.

👆 If it's not against your principles, you can let him hear the audio from pornographic films in the background.

When using lubricant, accentuate its sound when squeezing it out of the container or rubbing your hands together.

To heighten his auditory experience, blindfold him!

## The Visual Lover

As the name denotes, the visual lover likes to see what's happening.

When caressing him:

Let him admire you.

Wear erotic lingerie, outfits or accessories.

Some men are excited by specific body parts. Highlight them!

If it's not against your principles, let him watch pornographic movies while you caress him.

It's preferable to caress him in ambient lighting rather than in the dark so he can see you and what you are doing to him. Electric light dimmers or candlelight can help create an erotic atmosphere.

Caress yourself in front of him.

## The Oral Lover

Some men are crazy about oral experiences, such as kissing, licking or sucking, activities which amplify the intensity of their sexual experience.

When caressing an oral lover:

☞ Let him lick and nibble at you.

☞ Learn what he likes to have in his mouth and spoil him!

☞ Incorporate food in your sessions (whipped cream, chocolate, etc.).

## The Olfactory Lover

Some men are turned on by odors. Perfume, body odors, the smell of leather or latex can easily excite them even before you lay a finger on them.

When caressing an olfactory lover:

☞ Wear a sensual cologne.

☞ Use essential oils.

☞ Ask him what scents turn him on and infuse them into the air.

☞ Arrange it so he can smell your body while you caress him.

# And now... a few words about masturbation

You may have some considerations about masturbation:

> *"It's embarrassing!"*

> *"An adolescent activity..."*

> *"I have no idea how to masturbate him!"*

> *"For him, it's not as good as sexual intercourse or oral sex."*

> *"It's not proper sex, and it's a sin..."*

There's no shortage of uncomfortable notions about masturbation! Many of us still feel the awkwardness or shame about sexual pleasure we internalized when growing up from social and religious taboos. Some believe that masturbation is an immature activity and not fit to include in adult sex activities. Others may have religious considerations about it.

The truth is (as we all know) the vast majority of us have masturbated despite these taboos. Even after the sexual revolution of the past decades, some lingering embarrassment remains for many of us.

So let's clear the air: most people, and especially men, love to masturbate, and to be masturbated, if done well!

In fact, we have largely written this book about erotic touch to set you free from these negative and limiting considerations.

You and your partner need to give each other permission to fondle yourselves before and during any sexual encounter, as well as the freedom to fondle yourselves without necessarily continuing on to intercourse or other sexual acts. With this simple permission, you will likely develop greater intimacy and, as a result, a deeper and more trusting relationship.

Forget everything you've learned about masturbation and remember this: If it feels good and doesn't harm anyone, do it.

# Lubricants

The use of lubricants is optional and a matter of personal preference. Some men can only be masturbated enjoyably with lube and others prefer the experience "dry". Some like to start dry and then, at one point, to feel the silky, entrancing sensations of lube. As with all the information we present in this book, we suggest you ask what he prefers. We also suggest you experiment with him to find which type of lube feels best. You'll only find this out by trying and asking your partner for feedback.

There are five major types of lubricants:

 1. saliva

 2. oil-based

 3. water-based

 4. silicone-based

 5. pre-ejaculate (pre-cum)

Despite the common perception that lubricants are essential, the use of some gentle techniques on the penis without them can be exquisitely pleasurable, especially at the beginning of a session. The secret is to begin with slow and gentle movements.

Applying a lubricant in the middle of a session can significantly alter sensations, but not always for the better! But don't take our word for it — try them out for yourselves!

## Saliva

Saliva is one the most natural lubricants around, but the relevant properties of saliva (quantity and viscosity, or thickness) vary greatly between individuals and the moment. If your mouth is able produce generous quantities of thick saliva, lucky for you and lucky for him!

If needed, there are ways to increase the thickness and flow of your saliva. You can:

Bite the tip of your tongue, as some actors do to combat dry mouth associated with stage fright.

Drink orange juice or other acidic drinks.

Place a teaspoon of sweet almond, olive or other vegetable oil in your mouth without swallowing and swish it around.

### Advantages

- Always available

- Natural

- Produces great sensations (if thick enough)

## Disadvantages

- Dries rapidly

- Can produce unpleasant friction if insufficient quantity

- May sometimes have an unpleasant odor

# Oil-based Lubricants

This category includes oils and moisturizing creams. If you use oil, try to use edible oils, as they are more natural and allow you to continue safely onto oral activities if you so wish. We recommend sweet almond oil and olive oil.

## Advantages

- Longer-lasting

- Doesn't dry out

- Natural, organic oils are available

## Disadvantages

- Not suitable for subsequent contact with condoms

- Can stain sheets and clothing

- Almond oil can go rancid in time

⚠️ **WARNING!** Do not use oil-based lubricants or petroleum jelly if you will be using a condom as these products degrade the integrity of latex and can lead to breakage.

# Water-based Lubricants

The greatest advantage of water-based lubricants is that they can be safely used with condoms.

## Advantages

- Does not damage latex condoms

- Available in varying thicknesses

## Disadvantages

- Sensations can be less pleasurable than with natural secretions

- May have a disagreeable taste

**Au naturel!**

For lovers of natural products, here is an easy, economical recipe for a do-it-yourself water-based lubricant:

**Natural Flaxseed Lubricant**
*Bring to a boil **2 cups of water**. Add **3 tbsp. flax seeds**. Lower heat, simmer uncovered for 15 minutes. Filter through a sieve, discarding seeds, then continue simmering the liquid for 10 minutes or until liquid is reduced by half of original volume. Pour into a sterile jar and store in the refrigerator. Clean all utensils promptly as it may be harder to remove when dry. When needed, take small quantities and warm by rubbing between your hands.*

## Silicone-based Lubricants

Silicone-based lubricants have a reputation for being superior to water-based lubricants because they last longer. On the other hand, they can stain fabric and are very hard to remove. One possibility is to cover your bed with a plastic sheet and have at it!

### Advantages

- Can be used with condoms

- Long-lasting

### Disadvantages

- Stains sheets and clothing

- May have an unpleasant taste

⚠ Some lubricants have warming or cooling effects. Please be prudent with their use as some may desensitize nerve endings or irritate the skin of the genitals and anus.

## Pre-ejaculate

More commonly known as "pre-cum", this liquid is secreted from the urethra when the male is aroused. Its purpose is to lubricate the penis during intercourse and to neutralize acid in remnants of urine that may be in the urethra. Some men produce significant quantities of pre-cum, and some none at all. It's an excellent lubricant, having been made by nature for this purpose.

### Advantages

- Natural

## Disadvantages

- Some people don't care for the taste

- Some men don't produce enough or any at all.

## The Lubricant Progression

There is an ideal progression, or order of usage, of lubricants for manual caresses of the penis. We have found it is best to proceed in the following order:

1. dry (no lube)

2. with saliva

3. with other lubricant

⚠️ If you use saliva and the saliva dries, and you continue without any lubricant, the resulting tackiness can cause an unpleasant friction, resulting in a temporary desensitization of the penis.

💡 When using a lubricant, it's helpful to warm it up by rubbing it together between your hands. This will prevent any thermal shock!

# The Cock Ring

The cock ring is a useful tool that can help maintain an erection. It is basically a ring of leather, latex, metal or other material that encircles the penis and the scrotum.

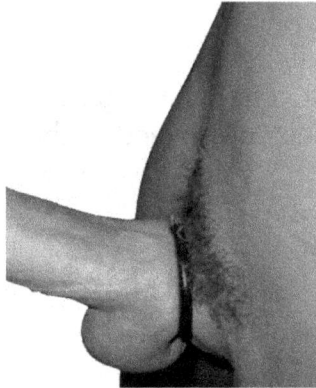

The cock ring circles the base of the penis at the top and the scrotum underneath near the perineum. Like a tourniquet, the cock ring constricts the blood flow leaving the penis, keeping more blood inside the organ and helping to maintain an erection. Many men report bigger and harder erections with a cock ring, and more powerful ejaculations during orgasm. It can also help to control the timing of orgasm, notably the ability to delay orgasm until desired, preventing premature ejaculation. A cock ring can also be used in conjunction with an erectile dysfunction drug for heightened effects.

⚠ Choose a cock ring size carefully. A cock ring should never be too tight. An overly tight cock ring can stop the flow of blood, and when tissues are starved of oxygen, they can die. A rule of thumb is that the cock ring should be loose enough to allow a couple of fingers through it when the penis is flaccid. If the penis turns purple when erect, or gets cold or numb, it is too tight. It could be dangerous to wear a tight cock ring for periods of more than 30 minutes at a time. Never sleep with a cock ring on. Having given all these warnings, it must be said, in all fairness, that a well-fitted cock ring is truly a wondrous thing!

# Hair, there, everywhere!

Another thing that will affect how your partner experiences your erotic caresses is the amount of hair that covers his genitals. For some, this can be a polarizing issue! Some people love naturally bountiful pubic hair, others really don't like it, and some have distinct preferences about how much hair is ideal. If you are going to be spending any time down there with your hands (or your mouth), chances are you have your own preferences. Although we don't get to control how much hair our body produces, we have the luxury of being able to trim or shave it. It should be noted that it is much easier to perform our techniques on the scrotum, anus, and perineum if your partner shaves his hair in these regions. In many demographic groups, shaving one's private parts has become very popular. This practice has existed since ancient Egypt and, no doubt, long before.

Is your partner open to the idea? You might offer to shave these body parts, which can turn into some awesome sex play! For men, the sensation of fingers or tongue on a shaved scrotum, perineum or pubis is completely different than with hair, as hair can mask the nerve endings in the skin. Having lots of pubic hair is almost like wearing clothes! For him, a good comparison is the difference in sensation between having his face touched when bearded versus when freshly shaven. For many, caresses performed on hairless skin are much more enjoyable.

It's a "Wow!" factor that every man should try to experience at least once in his life.

⚠ Shaving skin can produce tiny, almost invisible cuts. If you do not know the health status of your partner, it's best to wait a few hours after shaving to help prevent the transmission of any blood-borne diseases. As well, if there are any open cuts, both of you should make sure there is no contact with the other person's body fluids or mucous membranes. Always play safe!

# Strike a Pose!

Here are the basic positions in which you can perform our techniques:

**LYING IN BED**: Your partner is lying on his back with his legs extended, or knees bent. Position yourself on your knees between his legs or on your stomach. If his knees are bent, he can widen them, or he can let his knees fall to the sides. To ensure his comfort, place a pillow under each of his knees. This position gives you good access to his genitals and his perineum. You can also place a pillow under his buttocks to lift up his pelvis.

**SEATED**: Your partner is seated on a chair. You are on your knees in front of him, with your knees on a cushion.

**STANDING**: Your partner is standing and either:

- you are sitting on the bed or on a chair
- you are on your knees on the floor

**ON HIS KNEES**: Your partner is kneeling on the bed. Lie on the bed on your back or on your side. This position allows easy access to many of his erogenous zones.

**TWO ON A CHAIR**: You sit on the bed or in a chair and your partner sits on one or both of your legs facing you. It's better if he has both feet on the ground to lighten his weight on your thighs.

**ON ALL FOURS**: Your partner is on his hands and knees. This position is excellent for all techniques focusing on his perineum and anus.

# And what about pornography in all of this?

Pornography, considered dirty and despicable by many . . . can be your ally! You may object to the idea of watching pornographic films. Many of these misgivings are justified by the questionable content in a great many of them. However, if well chosen, it can be one more useful way to bring your partner to ecstasy.

It's possible you may feel jealous or threatened by the fact that he's sexually aroused by watching others. Know this: it's not because you're inadequate or not sexy enough. And it won't give him the urge to leave you for greener pastures.

The simple biological truth is there's nothing more sexually exciting for a man than novelty. Knowing this, you can turn it to your advantage. Use it as a part of your erotic toolkit.

Watching porn may bother you at first. Try it and see if you can gradually expand your comfort zone. That being said, do not give him permission to view pornography every time you have sex. There is a time and a place for porn. An ever-widening range of films is available. Pick out those that you do not consider degrading or offensive.

> **The last word**: Let him watch pornography if you want to double or triple the power of your hands. However, retain control over the choice of films and the on-off switch!

# Pay Attention!

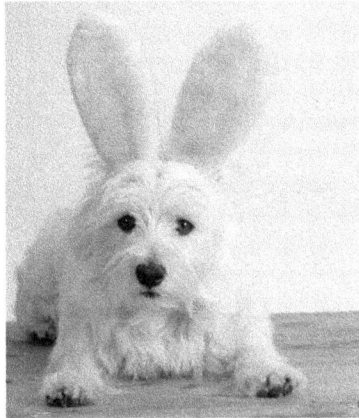

Because every man is different, you'll need to adjust your style to their tastes. To do this, the best strategy is to test the techniques with him to see which he prefers. As you already know, most men are not very talkative. So you'll need to use different methods to find out what he likes best. To help you in this process, we offer 5 winning strategies.

## ☝ Listen to the sounds he makes!

Listen to the sounds your partner makes when using a technique. It may be moaning, grunting or sighing. It can sometimes be difficult to tell the difference between the sound of pleasure and of pain. It's important to check with your partner to ensure it's all good.

## ☝ Observe his bodily reactions!

Observe your partners' body language. Here are some signs that let you know you're moving in the right direction:

- His penis is erect

- His erection bobs, twitches or pulses.

- His scrotum is firm and contracted (his testicles don't hang low)

- His respiration is rapid

- He spreads his legs apart

- He moves his pelvis

- He grimaces or smiles

**Feedback**

### Ask him!

There's nothing like having a frank discussion to find out what he likes. Unfortunately, as many men are reluctant to talk about this, we suggest you ask him to participate in an experiment. Try out the different techniques described later in this book and ask him immediately for his feedback on each. Since it feels a bit like an (inappropriate) medical exam, people who like role-playing games can use this opportunity to slip into their doctor/nurse uniforms!

Instead of asking him: "Do you like this?" which will usually lead to a positive but imprecise response, we suggest instead to ask: "How would you rate this technique on a scale of 1 to 10, with 1 representing little or no effect and 10 being outstanding?" When trying each technique, take the time to vary the parameters. It's important to note that the same technique can jump from a 1 to a 10 by changing the degree of pressure, using a different pace or changing any of the factors previously mentioned. This will give you a much better idea of what he likes and dislikes. We suggest playing this game for about ten minutes during foreplay. It will allow you to establish better communication in a way that's fun and exciting. And it's quite possible that this improved communication will be transferred to other areas of your relationship.

You can also ask very specific questions. Ask him if he likes precise movements. For example, "Do you like when I move your erection to the left and to the right?" You can get a lot of useful information. It may sound obvious, but it's surprising how many people are afraid to ask.

Do not be discouraged if, at first, your partner gives you results that never exceed 5 or 6, even with all the techniques in this book. You'll need to experiment with techniques and make adjustments such as varying the frequency or pressure. Initially, he may not appreciate a technique, but once you change the rhythm or pressure, it could become a favorite. You also need to know if he likes his caresses faster or slower, softer or firmer, and when.

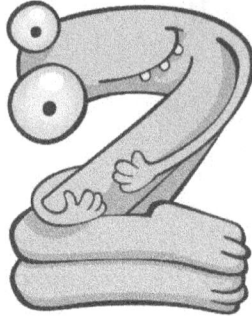

## ☝ Ask him to show you!

Since a picture is worth a thousand words, there's nothing better than a hands-on demonstration to show you exactly what he likes. Ask him to masturbate in front of you. Some men might be reluctant. Indeed, it's a very intimate activity. Encourage him to do it, even if it means that you also do it at the same time (but pay attention to what he's doing). You can learn how to push his pleasure buttons much more adeptly by knowing how he masturbates, the rhythms and speeds he uses, and where he likes to touch himself. Does he have other ways to do it? If yes, ask him to show you. Observe and make mental notes of everything he does, particularly the following:

- Where exactly does he hold his penis with his hand?

- What kind of pressure does he exert?

- Where does he place his thumb? Where are his fingers?

- What parts of his hand are in contact with his penis?

- How fast does he move his hand?

- How far does he move his hand up the penis? How far down?

- Does he sometimes pause? If this is the case, how long are the pauses?

- What does he do with his other hand?

- Does he change his pace?

- In which position(s) does he like to masturbate?

### Read this book with him

If you feel comfortable doing so, show this book to your partner and ask him to choose which techniques he would like to try with you. You might see the smile of a kid in a candy store. Your partner will likely feel privileged that you're taking the time to study the art of giving pleasure and sharing these wonderful techniques with him. He'll enthusiastically anticipate the hours of pleasure to come from your hands!

# The Volcano's Edge

When most men make love or masturbate, ejaculation is their main objective. This can often happen quickly, within minutes or even seconds. When it happens more quickly than desired, we call it **premature ejaculation** and it's a problem that many have tried to resolve using creams and a multitude of other techniques. For others, a quick ejaculation might seem perfectly normal. This latter group has yet to discover that sometimes the important thing is not the destination but the journey.

All men stand to benefit from experiencing a sexual practice called **edging** that consists of repeatedly bringing him to the brink of orgasm but without going over. Edging has elements in common with an ancient Indian practice called **Tantra**. One of many ideas behind Tantra is to experience profound sexual pleasure and spiritual sublimation without orgasm. In brief, this involves stimulating the sexual organs to almost the point of orgasm, and then stopping, or squeezing the penis firmly, to prevent ejaculation. It's quite possible to reach altered states from practicing this for an hour or more.

What should you do when you sense your man is approaching orgasm? This probably depends on how much time and energy you have. Most people just let orgasm happen.

To increase your partner's pleasure, we suggest you delay his orgasm. In order to get a better handle on the situation, you'll need some advanced warning of when he is about to come. Here are some helpful tips:

• His breathing may change.

• If he is masturbating himself, his tempo may change. Some men slow down a bit just before coming.

• His body may tense up.

• His scrotum contracts.

• His toes curl.

• His eyes may flutter, roll up, or close.

• He may grimace.

• He may grunt or make other guttural noises.

If he is silent and self-controlled, you may not see any warning. In this case, you will have to ask him to tell you when he is about to come.

## And then what?

Good question! You'll need to decide if you want him to come, or you want to prolong his pleasure. If you want to keep him on the edge of coming:

☞ Stop stimulating him (and prevent him from stimulating himself) for 15 to 60 seconds. Then start again, until he is once more on the verge.

☞ Squeeze the penis by surrounding it with your hand. This prevents ejaculation in some men. Be careful – avoid using too much pressure!

☞ Blow hard on the penis (with your breath). It's a trick that works for some men.

Repeat until he can't take it anymore or you run out of time!

# Orgasm

If your partner is on the brink of orgasm and you want him to have it, here are some points to remember: Don't stop! And don't change what you're doing unless he tells you (or otherwise indicates).

☞ Keep up the same movements, the same pressure and tempo. Keep going during ejaculation and for up to 15 to 30 seconds afterwards. Changing or stopping your movements too early during orgasm can make him feel like he is being robbed of his favorite thing, and that can be very disappointing! Some men do prefer a change in tempo, but only they will know exactly what they want. If your man takes the situation in hand, stroking his own penis, that's normal. Don't be offended. He just wants a perfect finish.

☞ Starting a minute after the end of ejaculation, the penis can become oversensitive to touch. Rubbing it beyond that can actually be unpleasant.

☞ If you had previously inserted a finger into his anus, remove it very slowly and gently a few seconds after orgasm.

# About those precious moments afterwards...

You've so far spent a lot of time exploring his anatomy. You've prepared an intense repertoire of sexual techniques for him. You've reviewed the pitfalls to avoid. You're ready to give him an unforgettably torrid night. The time comes. You use all the magic your fingers can conjure on him. He's moaning with pleasure, thrashing around, begging you for more, not to stop. He's putty in your hands. After a long, hot session, he can't hold back any longer and he experiences a mind-blowing orgasm. And then...

...he rolls over and falls asleep. Or gets up and decides he has to leave. Or sends a text message on his phone as he's raiding the fridge.

You're crestfallen. You were expecting more: an orgasm of your own, or maybe just a little appreciation, a moment of gratitude, or just some time cuddling, a little intimate pillow talk...

What happened?

His biology kicked in. While it's true that some men are interested only in their own pleasure, a part of his response is rooted somewhere in evolutionary biology. While we are not here to pursue that line of inquiry, we need to know at least that we shouldn't take it personally, or at least not totally. This is simply what many men feel compelled to do as a result of what we believe are hormonal and neuro-chemical changes in the body following orgasm.

A man's post-orgasm behavior can be modified through communication and negotiation. Some men will never change. Hopefully, this will not be the case for your partner. Certainly with age, many men become more considerate lovers. So if you can't get the reaction you want now, rest assured that, in most cases, time is on your side!

# For Best Results

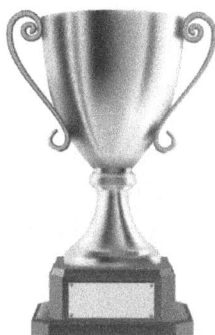

## 1. Take your time

There are good reasons for engaging in foreplay. Sexual arousal is not an on-off switch and most people need to warm up gradually. Avoid diving for the penis immediately. Let his anticipation and lust build as you stoke his desire with light caresses on different erogenous parts of his body.

## 2. Work with an erect penis

Most of our techniques work best when your partner is erect. Some of them may appear odd if he is not already aroused, and may have no effect.

## 3. Variety

It's a cliché, but only because it's true: variety is the spice of life, and nowhere is it more true than in giving sensual pleasure. Each technique can be performed in a multitude of variations. Indeed, by varying one parameter (the speed, rhythm, pressure, etc.) your partner will feel new sensations. He'll think that you have an endless range of techniques and will rejoice all the more!

Performing the same one, two or three techniques on a guy can become monotonously dull for the both of you after a while. On the other hand, being able to apply three, four or five different types of caresses to each erogenous zone is like treating him to a buffet. Stimulating some areas, and giving other areas a rest (and allowing their nerve endings to recharge) can be one of your most powerful secrets and will help to define your own particular style. But don't change too quickly; let him enjoy each maneuver for at least a little while!

## 4. Learn what he loves

You'll soon learn what caresses and techniques he likes best. You can perform these for longer periods, or use them skillfully to bring him to the edge of orgasm.

## 5. Be sensual

Be sensual, smooth, steady. Avoid jerky movements at first, though these can be exciting later on in the session. Add in other movements, like rubbing your body against his, kissing his neck, nibbling his nipples, caressing the inside of his thighs... Avoid chaotic tempos: stroking his penis quickly, then slowly, then quickly again can sometimes be irritating. If you want to slow down your tempo on a given area, give it a rest for a few minutes by caressing other areas, then move back. Conduct a symphony, not a cacophony.

## 6. Have a plan

Bring him to the edge of orgasm, and keep him there without going over, until you want him to. For him, nirvana is as simple as that!

## 7. Location, location, location

It's important to have a good understanding of how each erogenous zone responds to different kinds of stimulation. Since everything is connected to everything else, we highly recommend you read the Anatomy section, if you haven't already, so you can hone each technique to perfection.

## 8. Adjust for his anatomy

Adjust your techniques to his anatomy. The presence or absence of a foreskin should guide how you handle his penis. For more about this, please see the section on Circumcision. Also, if his penis is smaller or larger than average, you will need to make the appropriate adjustments.

## 9. Be holistic

Most of the techniques and caresses in this guide are directed at a man's genitals. This doesn't mean we should ignore the rest of his body. Remember to caress him everywhere!

## 10. Practice makes perfect

Remembering the best movements, pressures and rhythms for each erogenous zone might not be easy at first. What's true in sports and other activities is also true for this erotic art: you'll need to practice in order to become more adept and spontaneous. After a while you'll be multitasking without getting your movements, rhythms and pressures mixed up. The more caresses you can multitask, the greater the pleasure you will conjure.

# Managing expectations to surpass them

Here are some helpful tips to help you get better results:

## ☝ First, manage your own expectations

Learning the erotic techniques in this book may take time and practice. Don't expect to fully master them at the first attempt. And don't be discouraged if your man doesn't moan and thrash around in ecstasy the first, second or third time. You might even feel awkward or clumsy. Don't worry, you've merely left your comfort zone. Everyone's gone through this brief phase.

Remember that your partner has had years of practice with touching himself! Despite this advantage, few men know their body really well. They usually have a limited repertoire of self-caresses they perform when they masturbate. The average length of a male masturbation is less than 5 minutes!

Here's another little secret we'd like to share with you: your partner has not taken a course or attended a training on the art of caressing; he is self-taught. Rest assured there are caresses and feelings he has never before savored. You'll be the one who opens up a whole new world of erotic sensations for him with the tools and techniques in this guide. No need for magic powers: your fingers are all you need!

# ☝ Every man is different

Each man is unique and herein lies the beauty of things. Your man will have his own likes and dislikes, his distinct qualities, sensitivities and physical traits that are different from those of every other man. It's not surprising that each man reacts differently to the sensations produced by the techniques you'll be discovering in the next section. This is especially true about things that get him excited and keep him excited. One of your most important tasks will be to discover his particular erotic profile!

# ☝ Each body part reacts in a different way

Every male erogenous zone responds in a different way to a given caress, owing to its sensitivity and the type of nerve endings, along with the degree of pressure you're using and other parameters. Through playful experimentation, you'll learn which are his favorite erogenous zones and how they like to be touched.

# ☝ His sexual responses are not determined just by your presence and what you're doing to him

There are a whole range of physical, psychological and emotional factors that influence how each of us responds to sexual actions and stimulus. The following diagram illustrates some of them.

## Sexual Response Factors

How his body feels (energy/fatigue, pain, muscle tension)

His mental state (anxious or relaxed)

His self-confidence and sexual self-esteem

Other things on his mind (work, family, friends, finances, future...)

His general health, fitness and nutrition

What you're doing to him: the pure sensory stimulation

The effects of smoking, alcohol, drugs

What he sees: the person he's with, fetish items, pornography

What he imagines: his inner fantasy at the moment

His libido that day

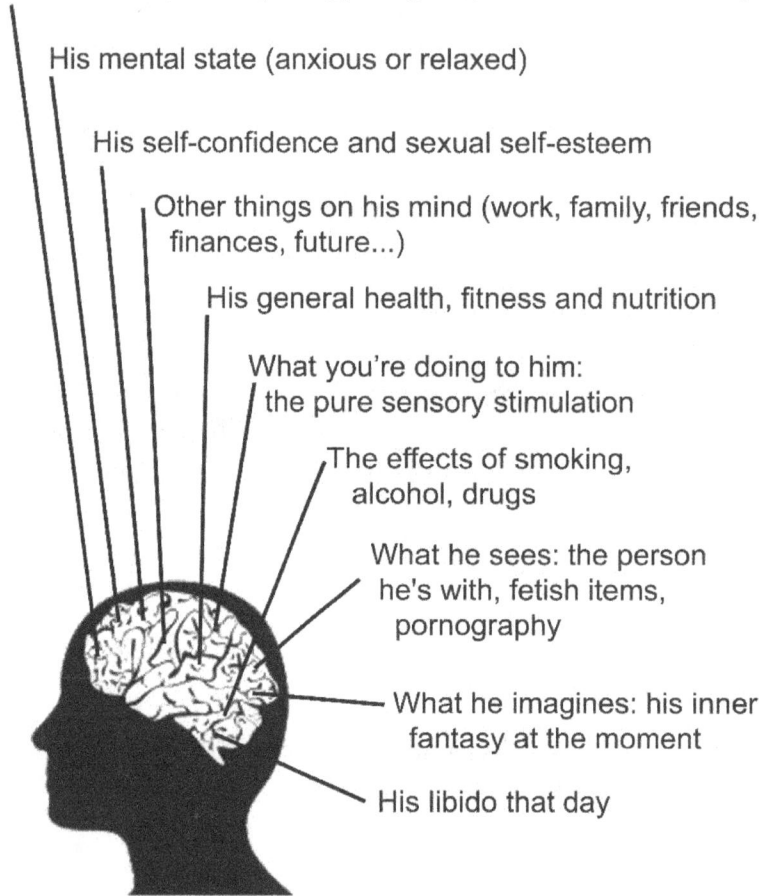

If you're not achieving the desired result, it's possible you need more practice or more feedback from him. However, it's also possible that other factors are at work. Some of these may be related to you, but as indicated in the previous diagram, many others factors are out of your control. What's more, the same technique used on the same person at two different times will not have the same effect, it's different every time.

# Faux pas

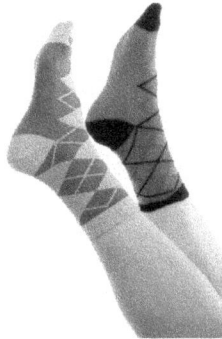

You may be intimately familiar with your partner's erogenous zones and have mastered some of the techniques in this book, but he might still have a disappointing experience and you'll never know why (because he doesn't tell you). Here, as a reminder, are pitfalls to avoid:

## ⚠ Dry, rough or calloused hands

They may not feel so bad to you, but to a sensitive penis that has spent most of its life sheltered by two legs, clothing and possibly a foreskin, even slightly rough hands can feel like sandpaper. Try using a lubricant on your hands, or latex gloves with a lubricant, or else carefully use the parts of your hands that are not rough. For best results, moisturize your hands daily.

## ⚠ Rings

Rings can scratch and pinch skin, and remember that cut precious stones have sharp edges. Take rings off before starting, if possible.

# ⚠ Nails

We've said it before, we'll say it again. Nails can scratch, especially up the bum. If you must keep your nails long and sharp, be extra careful!

# ⚠ Too fast, too soon

Starting with fast movements at the beginning of a pleasure session cheats both of you from the excitement of a slow, erotic build-up. Keep the big moves for the end.

# ⚠ Too strong or too soft

Gripping the penis too tightly, or too loosely can also lead to unsatisfying sensations.

# ⚠ Monotony

Always using the same few techniques or the same rhythms can be monotonous for your partner.

# ⚠ Erratic movements

While you should vary movements and techniques, too much variation in rhythm within short periods can be chaotic. Like a symphony, masterly caressing involves a progressive flow of coherent movements. Just think of how you'd like to be erotically caressed.

# ⚠ Focusing on one body part

As we saw earlier, focusing on one part of your partner's anatomy can create desensitization or irritation. Why limit yourself when there is so much to love!

## ⚠ Freezing at the wrong time

Orgasm is a result of the combination of your participation and his. If you suddenly stop what you were doing just when he's about to come, it's like dropping the ball at the most important moment. When you see he's close to orgasm, and you want him to come, keep performing the same movements with the same rhythm for at least one minute following orgasm, unless he asks you to do something else.

## ⚠ Talking too much

Better that we say it than he, right? Some people love talking during sex, and others dislike it immensely. You'll need to find out from him if he likes talk and what kind of talk (sensual, dirty, innocent, etc.) and you'll have to decide if you're willing to play along. But please be aware that too much talk can be distracting during erotic play.

# THE TECHNIQUES

And now, the moment you've been waiting for . . . the techniques! If you haven't read the first two sections of this guide, we highly recommend you do so, as their contents will greatly enhance your skills and confidence. If you have any anxiety about trying out the techniques on a real live man, we suggest you practice first on an object that resembles a penis. You can use an anatomically realistic dildo, which is the best approach, as it will give you a better idea of exactly where to put your hands and makes for a more solid learning experience (please forgive the pun). Otherwise, any phallic shaped object will do.

*In describing the techniques in this book, we've tried to be as precise as possible, and have often included the degree of pressure, as well as the duration of a caress. These are intended only as guidelines. Feel free to adapt them and to indulge your creativity and spontaneity!*

# CARESSING THE PENIS

*"I'm embarrassed to admit I'm not sure how to handle a penis…*
*I often have no idea if what I'm doing feels good or not."*
*- M.B.*

We've divided the techniques for the penis into two parts: basic and advanced. The basic techniques are those used most often by men when masturbating.

## Getting an Erection

Getting and maintaining an erection can sometimes be a source of anxiety for men, and indirectly for their partners. Many have told us that when their partner has trouble becoming or staying hard, they feel responsible. Unspoken thoughts hover in the air like: *"He's not turned on by me,"* or *"he's lost interest."* The pressure mounts to get an erection, feelings of inadequacy and fear of rejection may linger, and a vicious circle sets in. This is a not an uncommon occurrence.

Always remember: even though he might not have an erection, a man can still experience extremely pleasurable sensations when his erogenous zones are caressed.

Some men can get an erection looking at a carton of milk. If this is the case, take a moment to relish your good fortune. For others who may need more tactile or visual stimulation, and a little more time, here are some suggestions:

Avoid putting expectations and psychological pressure on him. If he's not getting an erection, it's possible he's not feeling horny, or he's tired. There are a thousand possible reasons!

127

Caress your partner's body without focusing on the penis. You want to avoid putting pressure on him to get erect, which can be counterproductive. Make your goal the sharing of pleasurable moments together, not the hardening of his penis.

Suggest that he touch himself. Sometimes, guys just need to start their own engine. Later on, while he's caressing himself, you can take more initiative and stimulate his other erogenous zones. Often, four hands are better than two!

Sometimes, stress and anxiety can interfere with getting an erection. A hot bath beforehand is an easy, pleasant and natural way to melt away tensions that cause blockages in the body.

Wearing a cock ring can help with getting and keeping an erection.

If you are both comfortable with the idea, using pornography (video, images or stories) can get things going.

Many men experience temporary or chronic erectile difficulties. Fortunately, there are many relatively safe prescription medications available that can resolve the issue. You may wish to encourage him to consult a physician to discuss the possibilities.

## Maneuvers While Caressing the Penis

A **maneuver** is an additional action that you perform while caressing. In fact, each technique is a set of maneuvers. We highlight some of these here as they can significantly augment the sensations felt by your partner while stimulating his penis.

☞ **The Facelift:** While holding the base of the penis with one hand, use the side of that hand or wrist to stretch the skin of the penis down towards its base by a few centimeters. This gently stretches the skin of the Heart of Pleasure. While stretched, lightly touch the Sweet Spot with the finger of your other hand. Intermittent touches can be quite pleasurable. This is a very subtle maneuver, so remember these two points:

• Stretch gently, not too much!

• Don't stretch the skin for more than 20-30 seconds. You can repeat as many times as he likes, but remember the pauses are as important as the stretches.

☞ **The Pubic Press:** while performing a technique on the penis, place the palm of your other hand on his pubis (above the base of the penis). Apply gentle to medium pressure, while gently pulling the abdominal skin in different directions.

# Techniques for the Penis

There are more masturbation techniques than there are men on Earth. Every man uses a few that he has adapted to his liking.

We'll start with the six basic techniques essential to your repertoire. Many men use them because they are very effective. Keep in mind that your partner might use techniques other than these.

We suggest you try each one and adapt them as desired.

# Basic Technique #1: The Fist Pump

1. Sit beside your partner.

2. Place your thumb on his Leverage Point and wrap your other fingers around his penis, as if you're holding an umbrella.

3. Move you hand up his penis towards the tip, until your fist encloses the glans and almost lifts off the penis.

4. Move your hand down the penis, to a point below where you started, without going further than what's comfortable.

If he's uncircumcised, his foreskin should slide over the head of his penis.

If he's circumcised, you'll reach the limit of the skin's elasticity, unless you're using a lubricant. Using the methods of rubbing or displacing the skin (described earlier in this guide) will yield dramatically different results. Try each to see which he prefers.

## VARIATIONS

☞ Start with a pressure of 1 to 2 on our scale. You can gradually increase pressure to 5.

☞ Vary speed and frequency by starting slowly and leisurely and then increasing each progressively, as you feel inspired by the moment.

☞ Change your starting position to higher or lower on the penis.

☞ Twist your hand gently as it reaches the head of the penis.

☞ Change the angle of the penis at the same time as you caress the penis so that it points lower (towards his legs).

☞ Caress his scrotum or his perineum along his Axis of Pleasure while performing this technique.

# Basic Technique #2: The Front Fist

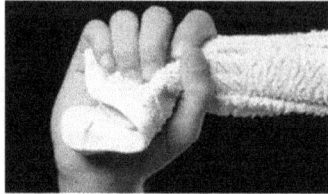

This technique is much like the previous one. The main difference is that you are facing him, and so your hand is reversed. The difference may seem trivial, but the sensations are anything but!

1. Face your partner.

2. Place your thumb on his Sweet Spot and your other fingers around his penis shaft, as if holding an umbrella.

3. Slowly move your hand up towards the top of the penis, until your fist encircles the glans and has almost left the penis.

4. Lower your hand to beyond your starting position, but never go lower than his level of comfort.

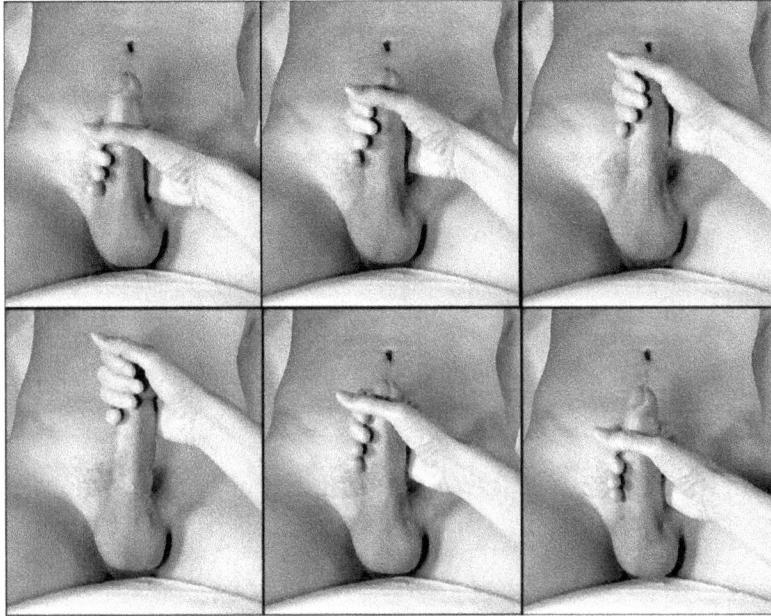

## VARIATIONS

All variations of the previous technique can be used here.

☞ Position your thumb upwards (pointing towards the head of the penis) at all times, so it can caress the length of the Heart of Pleasure.

☞ Perform the same steps above but use your index finger to rub the penis head.

# Basic Technique #3: Come With Me

1. Face your partner.

2. Place your thumb on his Leverage Point and wrap your other fingers around the penis shaft. You should be holding half of his penis in your hand.

3. Slide your hand up his penis towards the head, while rotating your hand.

If he's not circumcised, his foreskin should be sliding over the head of his penis.

If he is circumcised, you can try the methods of rubbing and displacing the skin (described earlier in this guide) to determine which one he prefers. This technique can be very pleasurable if your hand and his penis are well lubricated.

When your hand has almost left his penis, reverse the motion and the rotation, returning to your starting point.

## VARIATIONS

☞ Exert a pressure between 1 and 4 on our scale.

☞ Use a different starting point, either higher or lower on the penis.

☞ Gently squeeze the head of the penis when your hand arrives at that point.

☞ The variations outlined in the previous techniques can be integrated into this one as well.

# Basic Technique #4: The Sweet Treat

1. Place yourself either facing your partner or beside him.

2. Place your thumb on his Leverage Point and your other fingers (except your little finger) on the Heart of Pleasure. Hold the penis lightly.

3. Move your hand towards the head of his penis.

4. Move your hand back to its starting position or a little further down.

5. Repeat rapidly.


If he's not circumcised, try this technique with the foreskin pulled back, and also with it covering the head to see which way he prefers.

If he is circumcised, this technique works better using the displacing the skin method.

## VARIATIONS

☞ Exert a pressure between 1 and 4 on our scale.

☞ Start slowly, then increase speed and frequency.

# Basic Technique #5: The Virtuoso

1. Position yourself beside your partner.

2. Place your thumb on his Leverage Point and your middle finger on the other side, just below his Sweet Spot. Your index finger should be above his Sweet Spot but doesn't touch it.

3. Slowly move your fingers towards the head of his penis.

If he's not circumcised, his foreskin should slide over the head of his penis.

If he is circumcised, you'll arrive at the limit of his skin elasticity towards the head of the penis, unless you are using a lubricant.

4. At the end of the movement, move your hand back down, either by moving the foreskin down to its starting position or by sliding your hand over the shaft.

5. As you are moving your hand up and down, use your index finger to gently graze the Ski Runs, the Teaser and any other part of the Heart of Pleasure. As you become adept with this technique, you can increase the pressure exerted by your thumb and middle finger, while maintaining the lighter pressure applied by your index finger. Recommended pressure: 1 at the start and 5 towards the end.

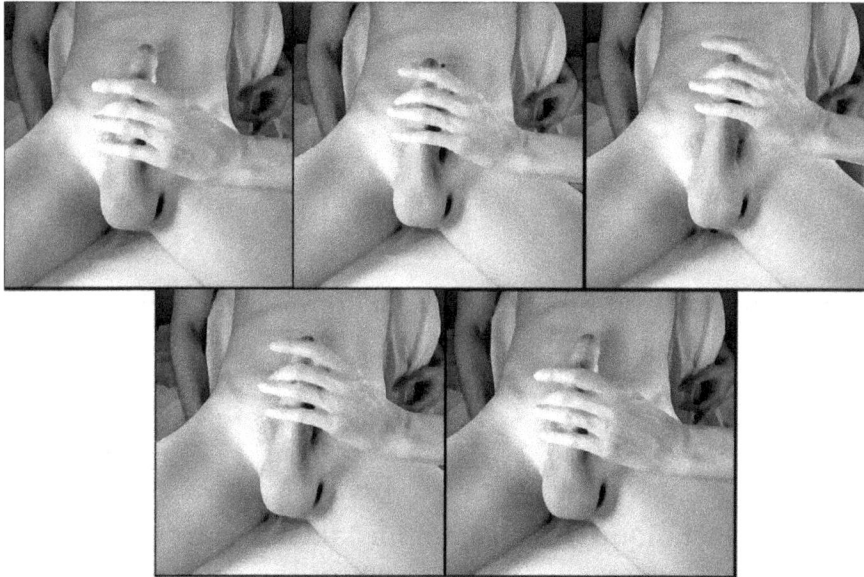

## VARIATIONS

☞ Vary the pressure applied by your thumb and middle finger, as well as your rhythm.

☞ Change the angle of his penis as you are moving your hand, so that the penis points down towards his knees.

☞ Caress his scrotum or his perineum while moving your hand.

# Basic Technique #6: The Jackhammer

Like a jackhammer that pummels into concrete, this technique can be very powerful. It's great for bringing a man to climax!

☝ This is a technique that some mistakenly start off with at the beginning. It should generally be reserved for the end of a session. Many men might not appreciate it too soon (it's the equivalent of a man who begins sexual intercourse with a woman by hammering away from the first penetration, without any foreplay).

1. Face your partner.

2. Place the palm of one of your hands behind his penis and encircle it so that the side of your thumb touches his Heart of Pleasure.

3. Move your hand rapidly up and down.

## VARIATION

☞ Perform this movement with your palm touching the front of his penis. You'll need to be beside him to do this.

☺ When performing this technique on a circumcised penis without lubrication, use less pressure. If you want to do it more intensely, use a lubricant.

# Thumbs Up!

We give a "thumbs up" when we want to convey our happiness and satisfaction. Here's a wonderful technique that reimagines this gesture and makes it even better.

1. Face your partner.

2. Position your hand, lubricated or not, as if you were going to shake hands. Gently wrap four fingers around the back of the penis. Place your thumb along the length of the penis in front.

3. Gently move your hand up and down the penis. Use a loose grip, so that your fingers do not constantly touch the penis, but intermittently touch or graze it at different points. You can exert a pressure between 2 and 5 on our scale.

4. Caress the Heart of Pleasure occasionally with your thumb.

5. When your thumb touches the head of the penis, you can randomly squeeze the penis gently with your whole hand.

Always begin this technique with a light pressure, and gradually increase it.

## VARIATIONS

Perform the same movement but gently change the angle of the penis, aiming it more towards his legs.

Perform this movement with a slightly trembling hand.

# The Magic Thumb

In this technique, your thumb wields magical powers and conjures mesmerizing pleasure for your partner.

1. Encircle the penis with all the fingers of one hand except the thumb. Your hand may be lubricated or not. Position your hand so that your thumb touches the Teaser. Your other fingers surrounding the penis should exert a pressure of about 4.

2. Keep your hand steady, and gently press the Teaser with your thumb with a pressure between 1 and 4 on our scale.

3. Move your thumb up and down, or from side to side, or in little circles.

## VARIATION

☞ As you perform the technique, change the angle of the penis by pointing it away from his belly and more towards his legs.

🔆 If your partner is very excited and hasn't ejaculated for a couple of days, this technique can trigger an orgasm.

# The Perfect Ring

When you want to convey that something is perfect, you might use this hand gesture, where your thumb and index fingertips touch, forming a ring. This is what your partner will use to describe the sensations of this technique!

1. Form a ring by touching your thumb and index fingertips. Lubrication is optional.

2. Place this ring around your partner's erection, close to the head of the penis.

3. Move your hand up and down, using a pressure between 2 and 4 on our scale.

If he's circumcised and you're not using lubricant, use less pressure. With lubricant, you can use a tighter grip.

## VARIATIONS

☞ Rub very lightly, just grazing (barely touching) the penis.

☞ Try exerting a little more pressure. In general, it's better to use less pressure on the Heart of Pleasure than elsewhere (but not always!). Try different ways and ask him what he likes.

☞ Starting with the ring around the penis at the coronal ridge (where the head flares out), make small, quick, light movements (of 1 to 2 centimeters, or half-inch) up and down, hitting the ridge repeatedly. We call this **Perfect Madness**. You'll see why!

☞ Starting from the base of the penis, as you slowly move up, gently squeeze and release the penis 3 or 4 times before reaching the head. The pressure should be between 2 and 4 on our scale.

# Double Rings

1. Lubricate both your hands if desired.

2. Form a ring with the thumb and index finger of your right hand. Do the same with your left hand.

3. Place one ring over the head of your partner's penis and begin slowly moving it down the shaft, with the second ring following close behind. The rings should be loosely touching each other, and you should be able to see your thumbs.

4. While keeping your thumbs in sight as much as possible, rotate each ring around the penis as they descend the shaft. Rotate the rings in opposite directions, back and forth. Use a pressure between 2 and 5 on our scale.

5. While performing the rotations, move the rings up the penis towards the head, and then descend again as before.

## VARIATIONS

☞ Allow both rings to linger a few seconds on the penis head and Heart of Pleasure while you rotate them.

☞ If your partner's penis is long enough, include your middle fingers, and if possible, add more fingers. The movements along the length of the penis will be limited, but the effect is awesome!

151

## Naughty Squares

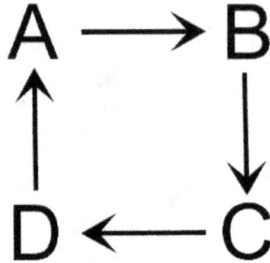

$$A \longrightarrow B$$
$$\uparrow \qquad \downarrow$$
$$D \longleftarrow C$$

We call this technique Naughty Squares because your hand will be drawing seductive squares around your partner's penis.

1. Face your partner while he has an erection.

2. Form a ring with your thumb and your index finger. Lubrication is optional.

3. Place the ring over the head of the penis and position it just under the corona so that the head is showing and your thumb is touching the Sweet Spot.

4. Apply a pressure of around 3 on our scale.

5. Rotate the ring 90 degrees to the right.

6. Keeping the same pressure, move the ring down by a couple of centimeters (1/2 inch).

7. Rotate the ring 90 degrees to the left.

8. Move the ring back up to its starting position.

9. Perform steps 5 through 8 as many times as desired.

## VARIATIONS

☞ Perform the movements with discrete, very square motions, or perform it with fluid motions. Pause for a second between each change of direction.

☞ While performing this technique, pull down gently on his scrotum, being careful not to overly squeeze his testicles.

# Polishing the Knob

1. Lubricate one of your hands.

2. Enclose the penis head with your lubricated hand.

3. Rub the head with your hand as if you were lovingly polishing the knob of a sword (an exciting metaphor) or a door handle (less exciting). Apply a pressure between 2 and 6 on our scale.

You can perform this technique with the foreskin either covering the head, or retracted.

## VARIATIONS

☞ With your other hand, perform the "face lift" maneuver which consists of gently pulling the skin of the penis down towards the scrotum.

☞ From time to time, move you hand all the way down the penis to its base.

# The Citrus Press

As illustrated above, a citrus press is a nifty kitchen gadget. If you've ever used one, you already have a good idea of the movement to perform.

1. Firmly hold the base of your partner's penis with one hand.

2. Place your other hand (lubricated or not) on top of the penis as if you were holding a lemon half.

3. Rotate the hand that encloses the penis head, as you would if you were reaming a lemon (but much more gently). Move this hand into closer contact with the head of the penis, so that the urethra (pee-hole) rubs against your palm. The fingers of this hand should caress the penis head, the corona and the adjacent shaft, including the Heart of Pleasure. Apply a pressure between 2 and 5 on our scale.

4. After a few seconds, slowly move the rotating hand up to its starting position. Then start again.

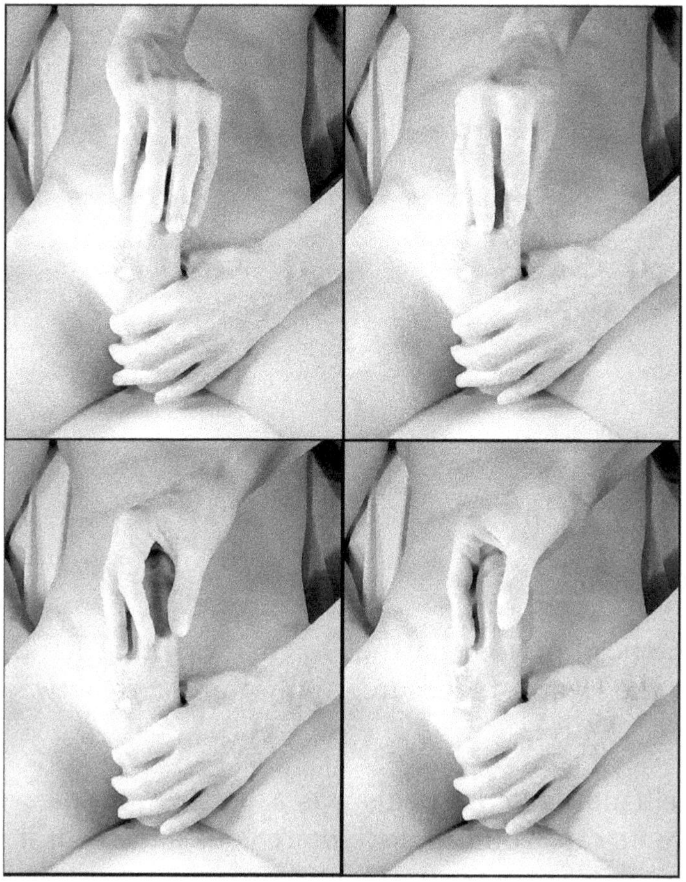

# The Bottle Opener

1. Lubricate one hand.

2. Encircle the head of your partner's penis with that hand so that your palm touches the Heart of Pleasure. Apply a pressure between 2 and 6 on our scale.

3. Move your hand as if the penis was a bottle and you were trying to gently remove its cap. You can also rotate your hand as if it were a screw cap.

## VARIATION

☞ Place your mouth on the penis head, as if it was the bottle opening.

# Playing the Flute

1. Place yourself beside your partner, who may be lying down or sitting.

2. Lubricate your hand (optional).

3. Place your thumb on his Leverage Point.

4. With the fingertips of the same hand, touch the front of the penis as if you were playing a flute, varying the position of your fingers. Apply a pressure between 2 and 6 on our scale.

## VARIATIONS

☞ Perform the technique with two hands.

☞ Place your lips on the head of his penis, as if you were really playing the flute.

# The Champagne Cork

1. Lubricate both your hands well.

2. Place yourself beside your partner.

3. Hold the base of his penis with one hand. Your thumb should exert a pressure on his pubis of between 4 and 6 on our scale. Your fingers should be wrapped around his scrotum, maintaining a gentle downward pressure (gently pulling the skin of the base of the penis and the top of the scrotum down).

4. With your other hand, encircle the head of the penis as if it was a champagne bottle cork.

5. Gently perform the movement you would use to ease the cork out of the bottle, but with much less force. Apply a pressure between 5 and 6 on our scale.

## VARIATION

☞ Usually when you open a bottle of champagne, you try to rotate the cork inside the bottle neck. Skip this step and while firmly holding the base of the penis with one hand, use the other hand to pull it up without rotational motion as if you were trying to separate the head from the shaft.

# One Way

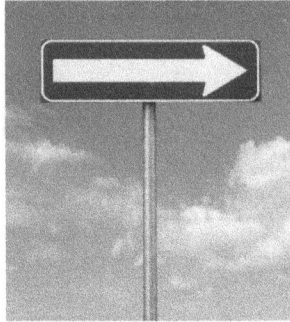

As its name implies, this technique involves performing a caress in one direction. You can experiment with different speeds, rhythms and pressures to discover the most pleasurable combinations.

1. Place yourself in front of your partner.

2. Enclose the base of his penis with one hand, lubricated or not.

3. Move this hand up the penis towards the head using a pressure between 2 and 3 on our scale until it is no longer touching the penis.

4. Pause for 2 or 3 seconds.

5. Repeat the movement a few times.

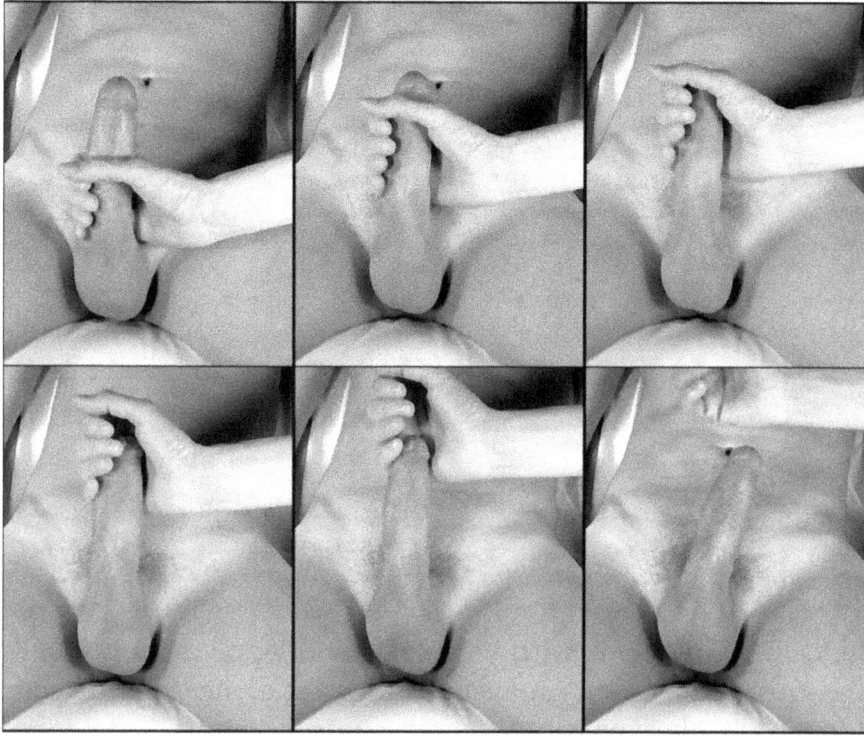

## VARIATIONS

☞ Perform this technique in reverse: bring your encircling hand down over the head and descend to the base of the penis. Warning: if your partner is not circumcised, proceed with caution as you are moving down so as to not go beyond his foreskin retraction limit.

☞ Use both hands, alternating right hand, then left hand. Each hand actually feels different.

☝ Your partner may beg you to perform back-and-forth motions or he may move his pelvis to achieve the same goal, because the sensations can become very intense.

# Unsheathing the Dagger

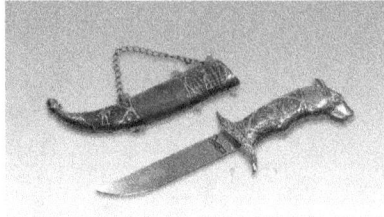

1. Face your partner.

2. Enclose the base of his penis with your left hand, applying a pressure between 3 and 6 on our scale. Your small finger and the edge of your hand should touch the place where the penis meets the pubis.

3. Configure your right hand in the same shape as your left, and place it around the penis in such a way that your index fingers are touching each other.

4. Move your right hand up until it leaves the penis, as if you were removing a dagger from its scabbard, applying a pressure between 1 and 6.

5. Keeping your left hand at the base, perform step 4 repeatedly with your right hand.

## VARIATIONS

☞ Invert the position of the bottom hand, so that your thumb is pointing down, touching his scrotum and perineum.

☞ From time to time, firmly squeeze the base of the penis up to level 6 on our scale. This will firm up his erection and make the movement more pleasurable. You can bring a great variety of wonderful sensations by varying the pressure, speed and rhythm of the upper hand.

# Go Bananas!

Making small circles with your index finger beside the temple of your head is a common gesture that signifies somebody is crazy. This is very similar to the movement that you're going to do in this technique.

1. Place yourself beside your partner.

2. Place your thumb behind his penis on the Leverage Point. Lubrication is optional.

3. Place your middle finger and your ring finger on top of the Sweet Spot, applying a pressure between 2 and 3 on our scale. Your index finger should not yet touch the penis.

4. Using your thumb and your middle finger, draw small ovals on the penis. The skin should move with your fingers. There should be an up and down movement as well. You'll notice that in doing this, your index finger rhythmically hits the front of the penis head as well as the Teaser. This is exactly what you're aiming for. Your partner will go bananas!

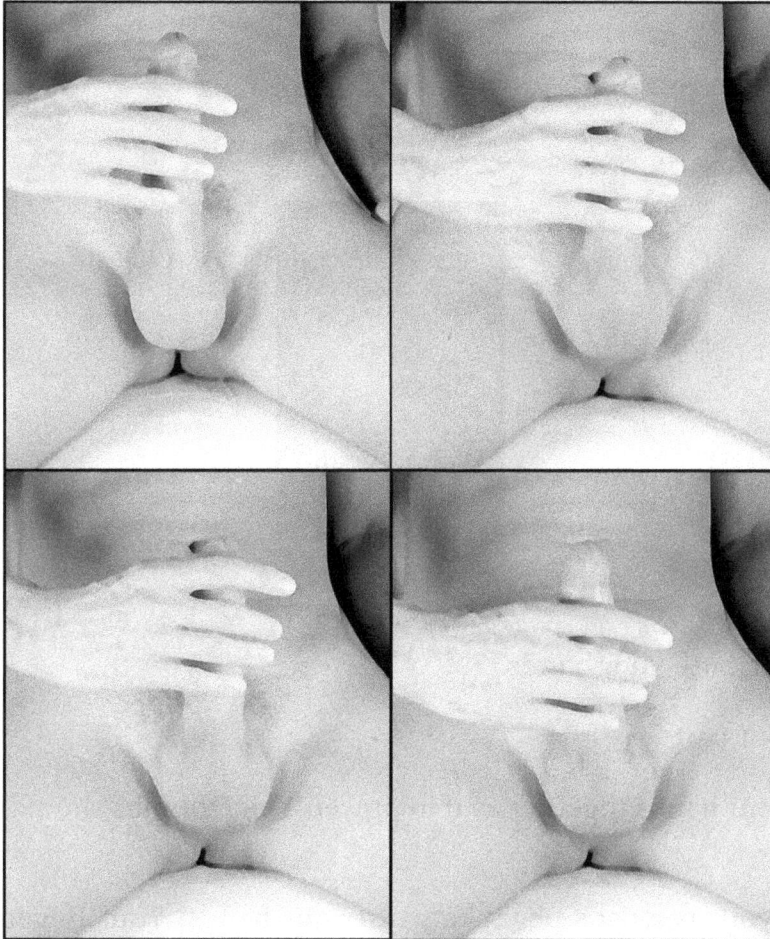

## VARIATIONS

☞ Do it in such a way that your index finger comes into contact with the Teaser, the Sweet Spot or the Ski Runs.

☞ Place your thumb on the Leverage Point and your index finger on the Sweet Spot and perform the movements, applying a pressure between 2 and 3 on our scale.

# I Beg You!

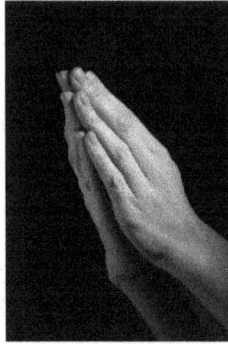

1. Lubricate both your hands.

2. Face your partner.

3. Place your hands together as if in prayer. Your thumbs should be facing you.

4. Insert your partner's penis between your hands. Your fingers and his penis should be pointing in roughly the same direction. With your palms, apply a pressure between 1 and 4 on our scale.

5. Slowly move your hands up and down the length of his penis.

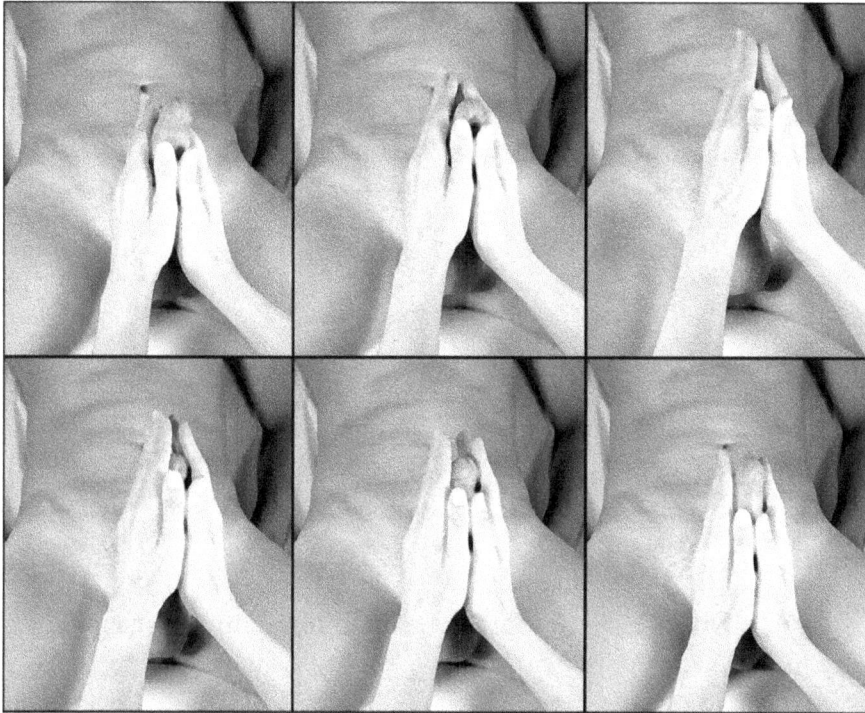

## VARIATIONS

☞ You can perform the same movement with space between your thumbs so that they caress only the sides of his penis.

☞ When your thumbs reach the Heart of Pleasure, you can pause momentarily and caress this region with your thumbs using a pressure between 1 and 3 on our scale.

# The Tower

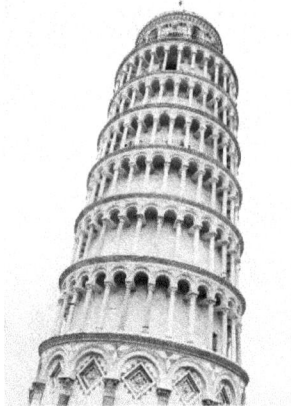

1. Place yourself beside your partner and place your lubricated hand in front of you such that your thumb is pointing down and the back of your hand is facing you.

2. Gently enclose this hand around his penis. The sides of your thumb and your index finger should be touching his pubis.

3. Gently slide your hand up the length of his penis.

4. When your palm reaches the head of his penis, continue the movement by wrapping it around the head of the penis and rotating your hand.

5. Slide your hand down, with your palm moving along the back of his penis. Your thumb should now be in front of the penis and your palm on the back of it.

6. When your hand arrives at the base of the penis, re-position it as in the first step.

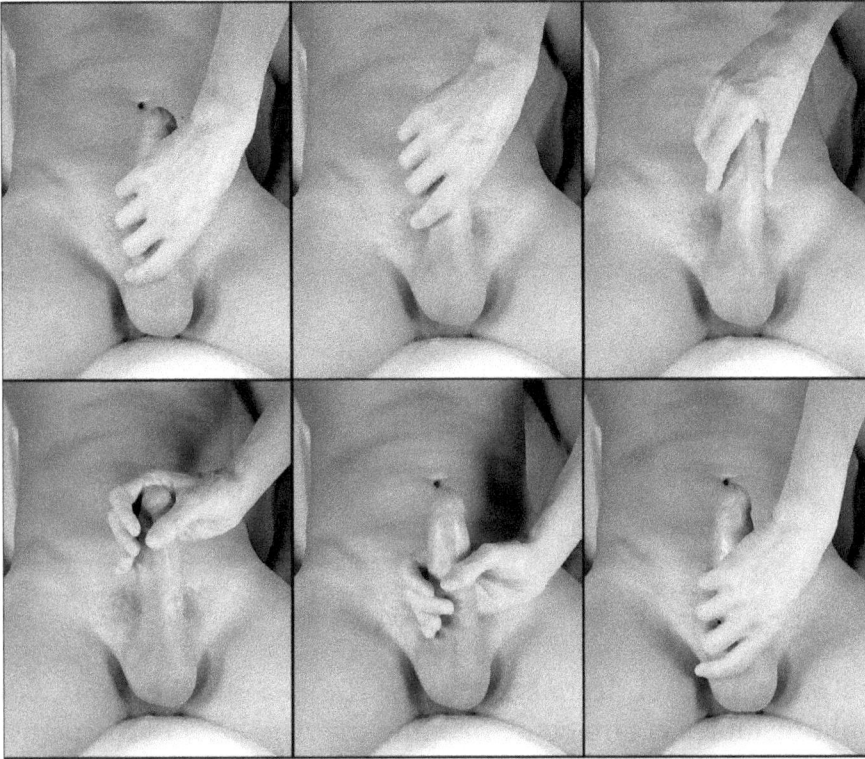

## VARIATIONS

☞ Once you've acquired some fluidity in this technique, you can apply it using both hands. In step six, instead of repositioning your hand, use your other hand to move up the tower. The hand that is "waiting its turn" can be used to exert a gentle pressure of pulling the scrotum down and away from the penis.

☞ Instead of repositioning your hand in step 6, you can bring the same hand back up, essentially reversing the movement. Pauses can add a lot of excitement to this technique.

☞ In step 4, don't move your hand down the back of the penis. Instead, open your hand and bring it down the front of the penis with your palm caressing it.

# The Ice Cream Cone

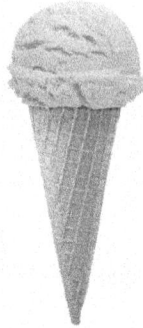

1. Face your partner.

2. Place one hand, lubricated or not, at the base of the penis as if you were holding an ice cream cone. Imagine that the head of the penis is the ball of ice cream.

3. Using the same hand, gently pull the skin in front of the penis down towards the testicles. If your partner is not circumcised, move the foreskin down as much as he can comfortably tolerate.

4. Gently run the index finger of your other hand, lubricated or not, over his Teaser.

5. Stimulate the Teaser for approximately 20 seconds and then pause for 10 seconds to allow his nerve endings to rest and recover their sensitivity. Then, do it again.

For those who like to incorporate food in their play, you can certainly use your imagination here!

## VARIATIONS

☞ In addition to the Teaser, run your finger over the other parts of the Ski Runs or the Heart of Pleasure.

☞ Explore a range of movements, from different fingers to your entire palm caressing the head and other sensitive areas of skin just below it.

☞ Instead of using your fingers or a hand, use your tongue! Lick the head as if it were a ball of your favorite ice cream. Stop to lick the Heart of Pleasure. Start with little nibbles, progressing to larger licks. Make sure you pause between each lick sufficiently to make him want for more. While pausing between licks, exert a slightly greater pressure on the base of the penis with your hand.

# Intertwining

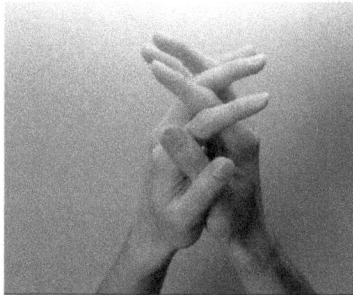

1. Face your partner.

2. Lubricate your hands.

3. Interlace the fingers of both your hands.

4. Place your interlaced fingers behind the penis. Your little fingers should be touching the point where the penis meets the pubis.

5. Place your thumbs beside each other in front of the penis. The penis should now be encircled by your hands. Apply pressure between 2 and 5 on our scale.

6. Slide your hands up the penis until your palms are on the penis head.

7. Slide back down.

8. Repeat.

9. Vary your rhythm and pressure.

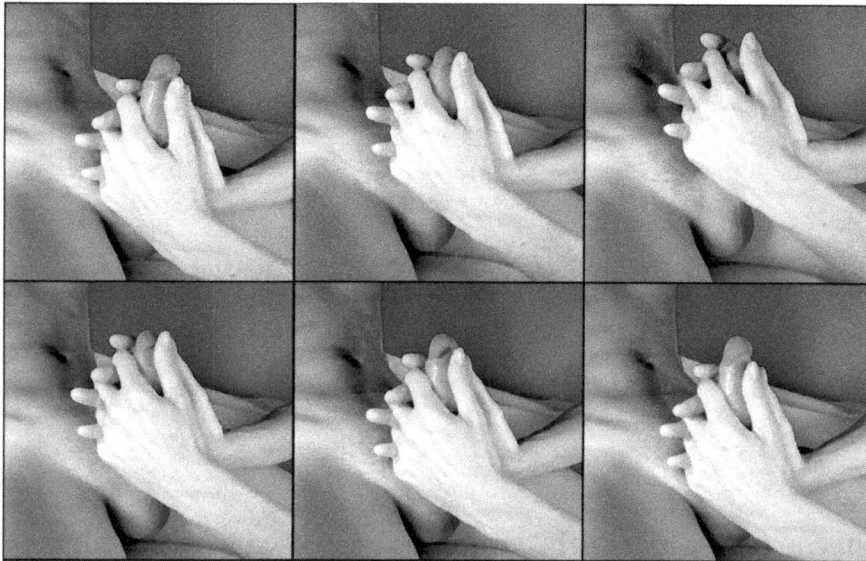

## VARIATIONS

☞ Exert greater pressure when your hands are around the head or at the base of the penis.

☞ When your palms reach the head, squeeze briefly with a pressure of 6 on our scale and then release.

☞ Rotate your hands around the penis as they go up and down.

# The Love Potion

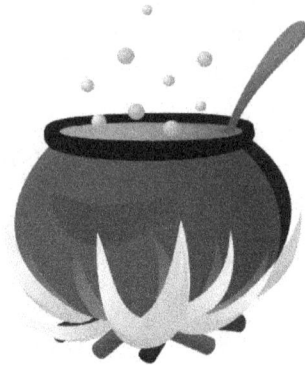

Imagine that you're a witch (a beautiful and talented one, of course) and you're brewing a love potion in your cauldron. This technique uses that stirring motion. However you won't need the wooden spoon — your partner's penis will be your utensil.

1. Your partner should be fully erect and lying on his back, or standing up.

2. With one hand, lubricated or not, gently take hold of his penis by the head. Exert a pressure of 2 or 3.

3. Draw circles with his penis head as if you were stirring a potion.

4. Stir a few times in one direction, and then in the other. You can vary the size of the circle, making sure you don't go too far.

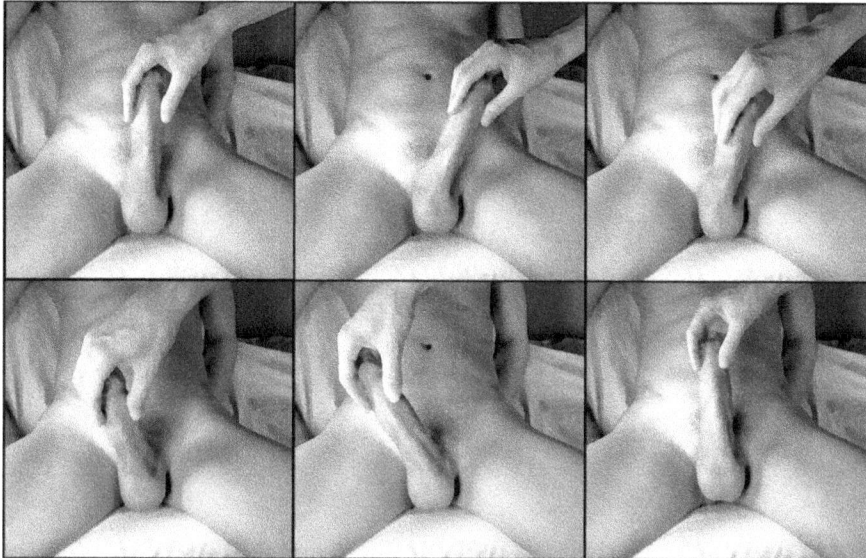

If you happen to be under the covers while using this technique, try allowing the front of the penis head to come into contact with the sheet in step 3.

## VARIATION

☞ Hold the penis at the Heart of Pleasure. Move the penis head around in circles, allowing the head to come into occasional contact with your lips. This resembles the motion used to put on lipstick.

179

# Squeezing the Straw

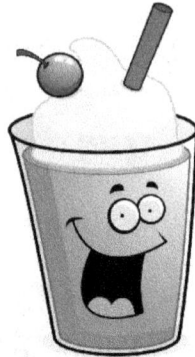

Until now, we've warned you against applying too much pressure on the penis. The following technique is the exception to this rule. Many men, but not all, find it very pleasurable.

1. Hold your partner's erection with your thumb and index finger. Your thumb should be somewhere between the penis head and the Leverage Point. Your index finger should be on the Heart of Pleasure. You can also use your middle finger, which should be placed beside your index finger.

2. Squeeze the penis as if you wanted your fingers to touch each other. Start with gentle pressure and slowly increase the pressure until you have a good idea of the limit between his pleasure and discomfort. Some men like it when you go up to level 6 on our scale.

3. Release.

4. Repeat every few seconds taking care to not rub or move the penis skin around.

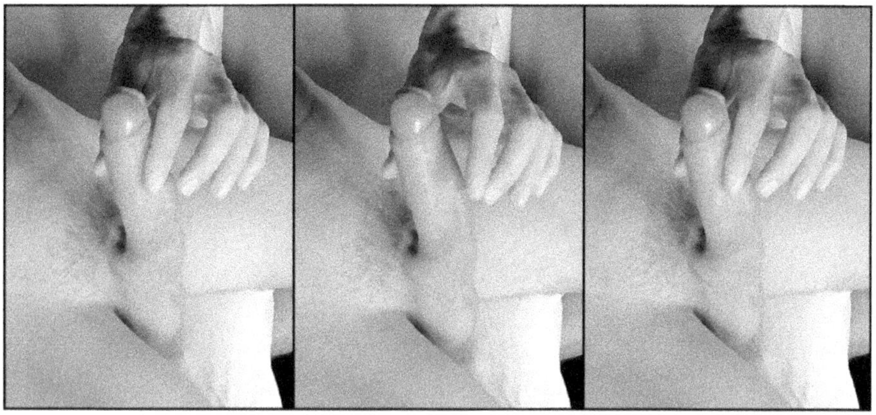

# The Fan

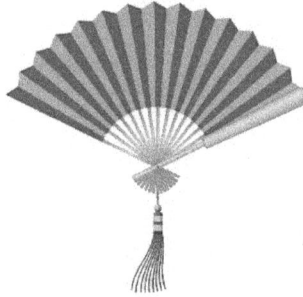

You have perhaps seen Spanish flamenco dancers masterfully manipulating a fan in their hand. This is the type of motion you want to reproduce.

1. Place yourself near your partner, who could be lying on his back or standing up.

2. Using one hand, lubricated or not, hold the penis at its base, applying a pressure of 2 or 3 on our scale.

3. Place the palm of your other hand in front of his Heart of Pleasure.

4. Use the hand at the base of the penis to move the penis so that it taps the palm of your other hand. Start with taps of pressure level 3 and slowly increase pressure to see how much he likes best.

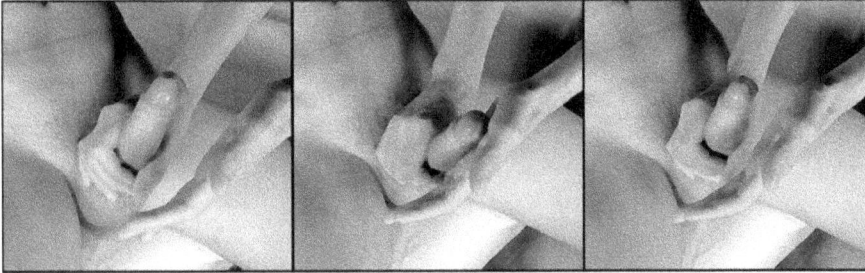

## VARIATIONS

☞ In step 4, replace your hand with your tongue.

☞ Rub his penis around the palm of your lubricated hand.

☞ Try gently slapping the penis against other surfaces. Use your creativity!

# CARESSING THE SCROTUM

For some men, having their balls caressed while their penis is being stimulated can be a mind-blowing experience. For the following techniques, it's essential that your partner has a full erection. It's best to wait until this happens in your play session before attempting these techniques.

Be careful! Testicles are **very** sensitive to pressure. Treat them gently. In fact, it's not the testicles that you're trying to caress directly but the scrotum, the sensitive skin that surrounds them.

All the techniques presented in this section have the potential to be ticklish for your partner. If this is the case, you can try them with slightly more pressure, and using your entire hand instead of just a few fingers. You could also begin with a full hand and then try fewer fingers later in the session when he's gotten used to the sensations.

# Infinite Pleasure

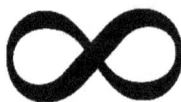

∞

You may be familiar with the mathematical symbol for infinity which resembles a figure 8 lying on its side. This is the pattern that you're going to reproduce on your partner's scrotum.

1. Place yourself in front of your partner in such a way that you have access to his scrotum. He can be standing, sitting or lying down.

2. Use your finger, lubricated or not, to trace the symbol of infinity on his scrotum, taking care to draw a circle on each testicle. Use a level of pressure between 1 and 4 on our scale.

☝ This caress must be done at the same time that his penis is being stimulated.

🔆 This caress gives more pleasure when the scrotum is contracted.

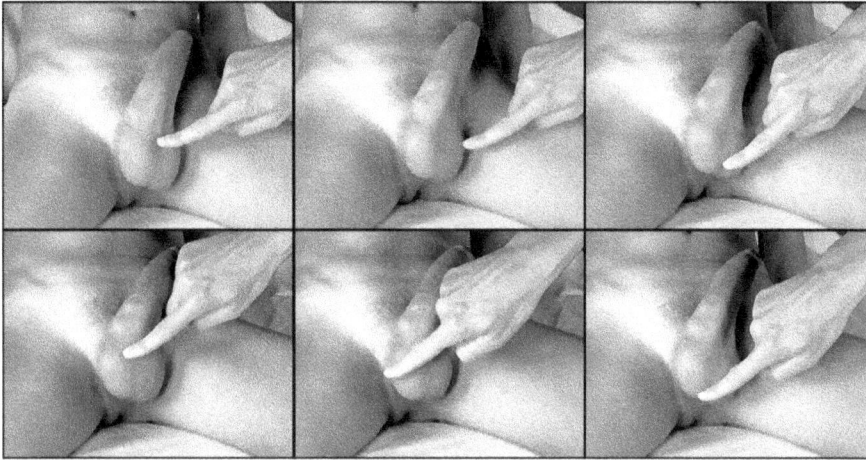

## VARIATIONS

☞ Perform this technique using your tongue.

☞ Follow the above steps but trace a bigger symbol and go further out towards the inner creases of the thigh and the perineum.

☞ Trace multiple circles on one testicle before moving to the other.

# The Octopus

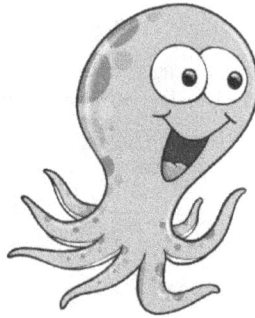

With this technique, your partner can experience the intense pleasure of receiving multiple caresses simultaneously.

1. Position yourself near your partner, who can be lying on his back or standing.

2. Place your hand, lubricated or not, in front of you, palm facing up.

3. Flex your fingers as if you're holding a grapefruit.

4. Place your fingers around his scrotum.

5. Move all your fingers independently, imitating the motions of the tentacles of an octopus. Delicately massage the skin of the scrotum with a pressure of 1 or 2 on our scale.

## VARIATIONS

☞ Your finger movements can be simultaneous, like those of a jellyfish bobbing in a current.

☞ From time to time, allow your fingertips to brush further back along the perineum.

☞ Move your hand downwards, which will allow your fingers to touch the entire length of his scrotum.

# The Tea Bag

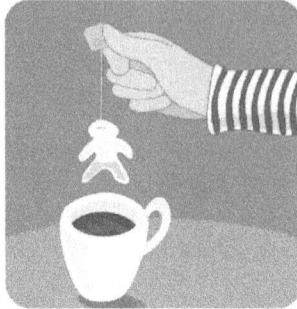

1. Place yourself in front of or beside your partner, who is standing or lying.

2. Using your thumb and index finger, gently encircle the scrotum between the perineum and the testicles. Lubrication is optional. The testicles should be hanging below your hand. Don't squeeze too tightly, just a 1 on our scale! This technique may be difficult to perform on men whose scrotum contracts tightly when aroused. In this case, try the technique when he is less excited.

3. Hold the position for a few seconds.

4. Gently pull the scrotum away from the body.

⚠ Don't squeeze too hard!

☝ Don't forget to stimulate your partner's penis at the same time!

## VARIATIONS

☞ Gently move the scrotum back and forth in a pendulum motion.

☞ Caress the scrotum with the fingers of your other hand or with your tongue.

## 👓 Did you know?

*Tea-bagging refers to the act of dipping one's testicles into someone else's mouth, as one dips a tea bag in a cup of hot water.*

# Take a Number!

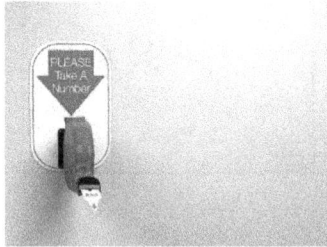

We've all been at a service counter and had to take a number from a dispenser in order to be served. This is the motion you'll be replicating, using your partner's scrotum instead!

1. Place yourself in front of your partner, who is standing or lying on his back.

2. Using your thumb and index finger, gently hold the skin at the bottom of his scrotum between his testicles.

3. Gently pull the scrotum away from his body. The scrotum should move at most 1 centimeter (a quarter inch). Use a pressure between 2 and 4 on our scale.

4. Pause briefly for a few seconds.

5. Repeat steps 2 to 4.

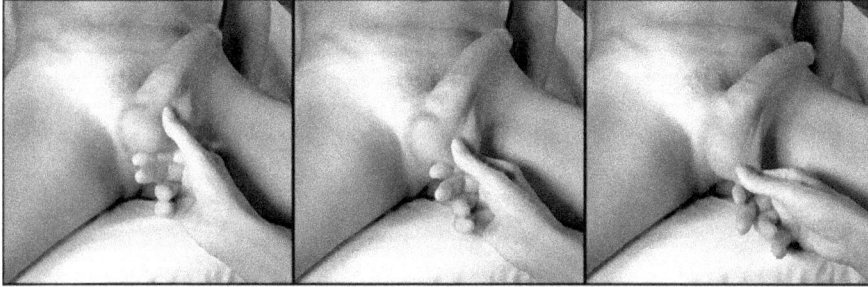

It's easier to perform this technique when your hands and his scrotum are not lubricated, as you'll need to maintain your grip without slipping.

As with all the other techniques involving the scrotum, this works best when his penis is being stimulated at the same time.

# CARESSING THE PERINEUM (AND THE INNER CREASES OF THE THIGH)

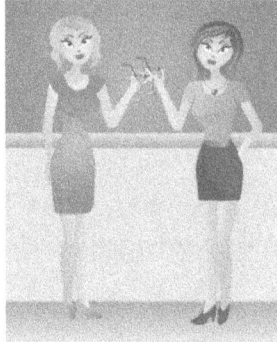

*"Greg called it his 'grundle'. Pete said 'perineum'."*
*"I call it the best thing since chocolate ice cream!"*

It's finally time to reveal one of the best kept secrets of male sexual pleasure: the wonders of the perineum and our techniques for caressing it. This can be extremely exciting for your partner. And it's quite possible that he has never been caressed there before.

Some men may find the perineum a ticklish area. In this case, proceed gradually, or try another time. The following techniques work best when your partner is lying on his back, with his legs spread apart, as this will give you greater access to the prized real estate. Even better if he bends his legs and you slip a cushion under his pelvis!

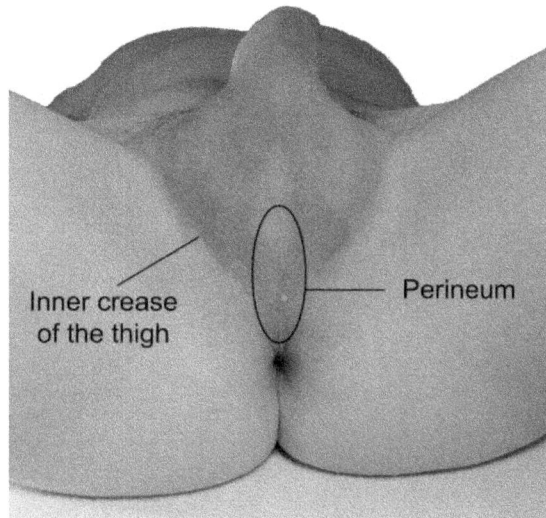

Inner crease
of the thigh

Perineum

Please note:

- He may find these caresses more pleasurable if his perineum is shaved.

- You may have to lift up his scrotum to gain full access to his perineum.

- The following techniques are pleasurable only while his penis is being stimulated at the same time.

# Holding the Bowling Ball

1. Position yourself beside your partner, who can be standing or lying on his back.

2. Position one hand, lubricated or not, underneath his scrotum, as if it were a bowling ball (without holes), and you were lifting it from underneath.

3. Slide your hand further back along his perineum. Avoid putting any pressure on his testicles.

4. Apply a pressure between 2 and 5 on our scale for a few seconds and then release.

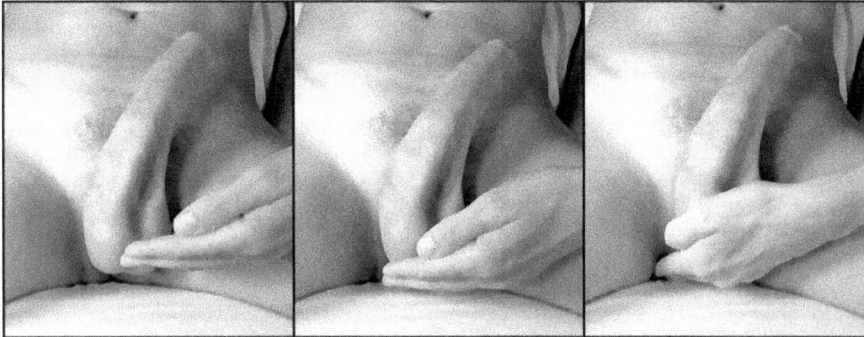

## VARIATION

☞ Move your hand further backward and forward, gliding it along the perineum. The feeling is usually more intense when your hand is lubricated, and you can proceed with faster movements.

# The Ski Hill

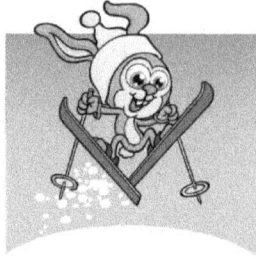

Alpine skiers can choose between skiing straight down or zigzagging across the hill. It's this latter pattern you'll be replicating in this technique.

1. Your partner is lying on his back, with his legs bent at the knees and spread apart.

2. Place your finger, lubricated or not, on his perineum near the scrotum.

3. Slowly move your finger towards his anus, as if you were skiing down a hill, zigzagging back and forth across his perineum. Apply a pressure between 1 and 3 on our scale. Take your time to go down the hill. This technique usually produces a lot of pleasure when done slowly.

4. Stop when your finger reaches the anus.

5. Repeat the movement.

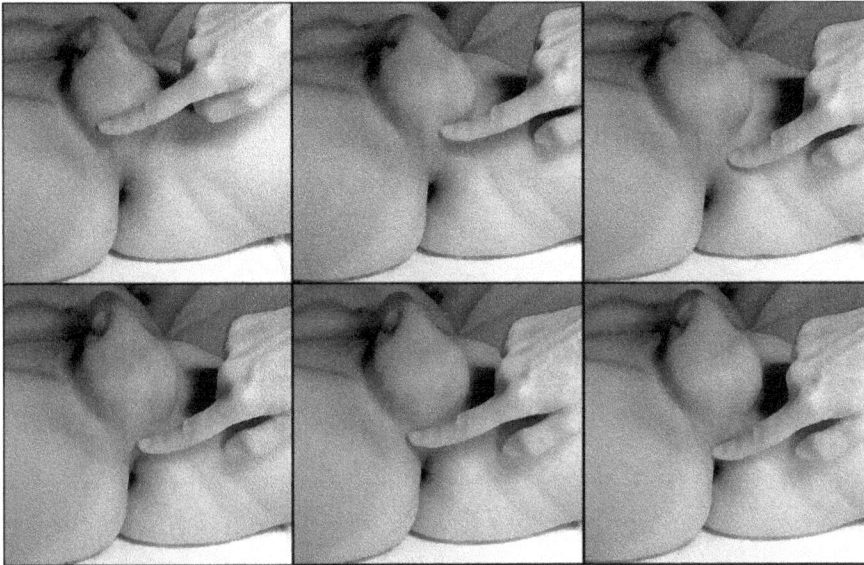

## VARIATIONS

☞ To produce even more spectacular sensations, use your tongue instead of your finger. To avoid neck strain, you'll need to lie on your stomach on the bed. You can slide a pillow under your partner's pelvis to give you easier access to the ski hill!

☞ Start from the bottom and perform the same movements in the opposite direction.

☞ This technique can also be performed when your partner is standing.

# Come Here!

You've no doubt used the universal hand sign to "come here". It's the same movement you're going to apply to the area where the perineum meets the scrotum.

1. Position yourselves so that you have access to your partner's perineum, who can be standing or lying down.

2. Place your index finger, lubricated or not, on his perineum, around 3 centimeters (one inch) behind his scrotum.

3. Move your finger towards his scrotum, using a pressure between 2 and 5 on our scale.

4. Repeat.

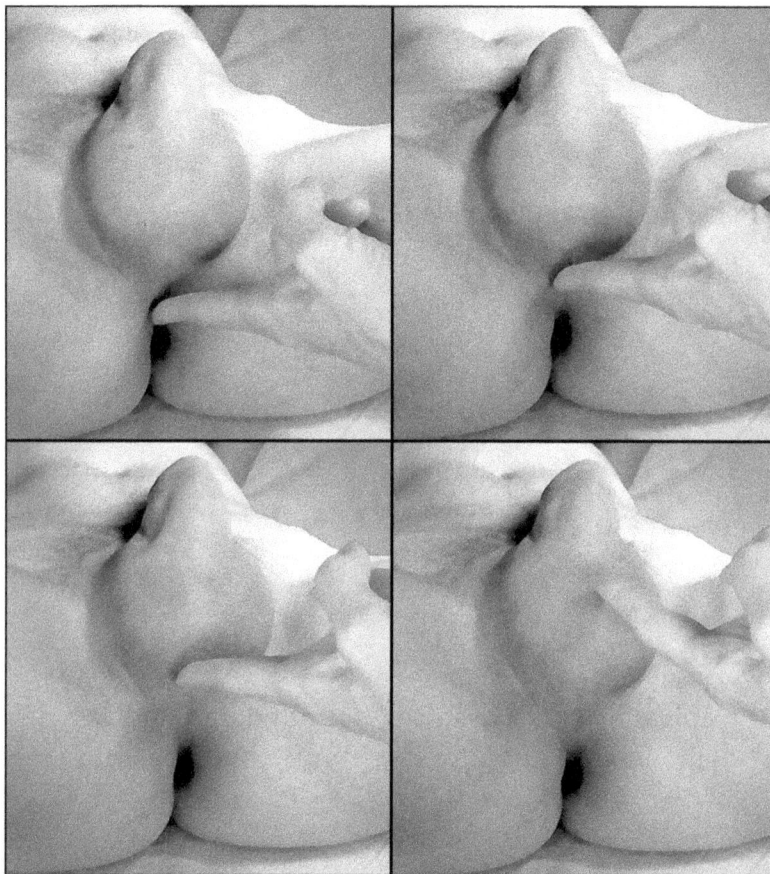

## VARIATIONS

☞ Double the impact of this technique by using both your index finger and your middle finger independently. Try one gesture with your index finger on one side of the perineum, then one with your middle finger on the other side and repeat, barely pausing between gestures.

☞ Perform the motion using all your fingers, except your thumb. Try using your fingers independently, and also try using your fingers together at once.

# Cayo Largo

**CAYO LARGO DEL SUR**

**Playa Paraiso**   **Playa Linda**

Cayo Largo... a tropical island paradise, bounded by endless deserted beaches. Inspired by this idyllic landscape, here is a simple but powerful technique that can multiply his pleasure by three.

1. While his erect penis is being stimulated (by you or by himself), gently caress the skin where the penis is joined to the body behind the scrotum. Using the map of Cayo Largo above as a metaphorical guide, aim for the area between Playa Paraiso and Playa Linda. If his testicles get in the way, you may have to delicately move them aside. If his scrotum is contracted, it will be easier to perform this technique.

2. Use two fingers to slowly draw circles or stroke the area from front to back, or back to front – the escalation of his pleasure should be quite evident. Make sure you are pressing on his hidden penis, and not directly on his testicles.

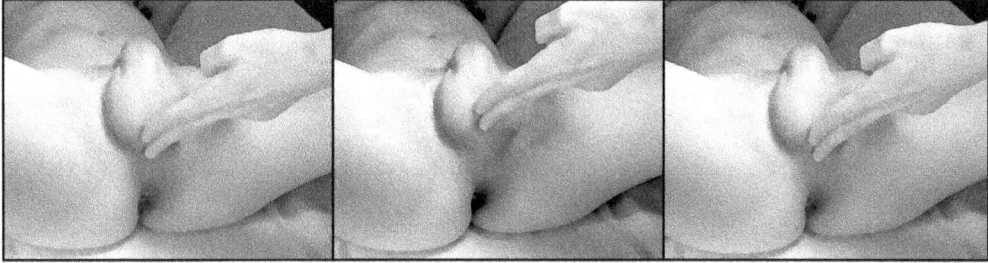

# The Toothpaste Tube

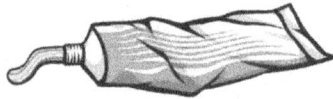

Imagine a long and irregularly-shaped tube of toothpaste that extends from the tip of the penis all the way to the edge of the anus. Actually, that IS the penis, including its hidden root. Pretending it's a tube of toothpaste can lead to very pleasurable sensations!

This is the image you need to hold in your mind for this mind-blowing technique where the "tube" is actually the hidden penis which sits above the perineum and becomes firm when the penis is erect.

1. Gently squeeze both sides of the "tube" with your fingers for a few seconds, then release. **Important:** apply pressure on the sides rather than directly upwards at the center, as this could be uncomfortable for some.

2. Move to another spot along the "tube" and re-apply pressure. In some areas, this gentle embrace can deliver jolts of sublime pleasure!

3. At the start, squeeze gently and then gradually increase pressure, as you would actually use on a real tube of toothpaste, between 2 and 4 on our scale.

⚠ Some parts of the perineum are more sensitive to pressure than others, particularly at the center. Monitor your partner's reactions or ask him for feedback to get a better sense of how much pressure to apply at each point along his perineum. Don't squeeze the testicles.

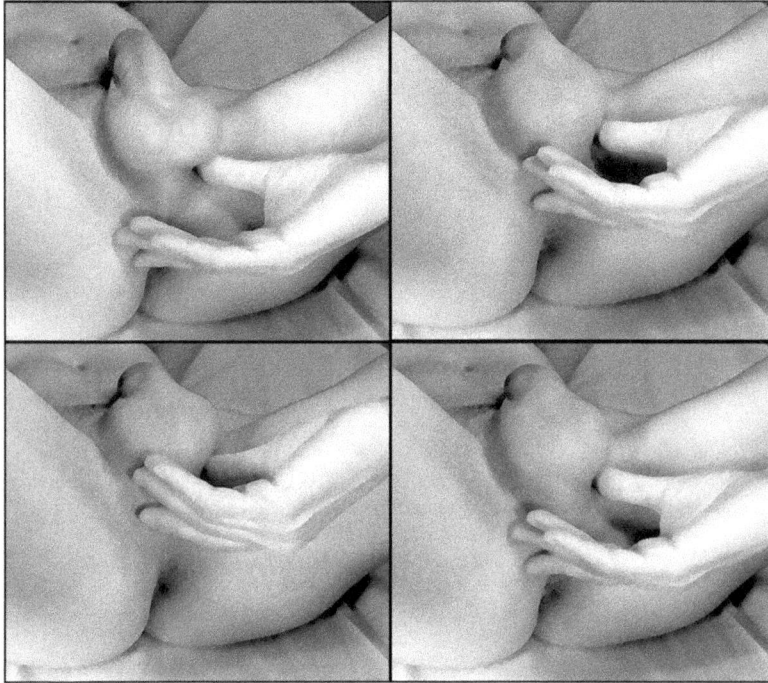

## *VARIATIONS*

☞ Apply the steps above using the fingertips of both hands. Try touching as many points as possible.

☞ Let your fingers drift to the inside of his thighs.

☞ Squeeze the length of his penis with your other hand. Apply this pressure from the sides of the penis rather than from front to back.

# Curtains!

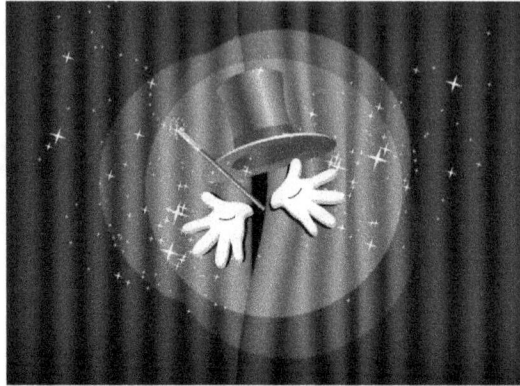

*Let the show begin!*

1. Position yourself near your partner, who is lying down on his back.

2. Place your fingertips (except the thumb) of one hand on the internal crease of one of his thighs. Lubrication is optional.

3. Slowly use your fingers to stroke across the perineum towards the opposite thigh, as if you were drawing back a curtain. Apply a pressure between 2 and 5 on our scale.

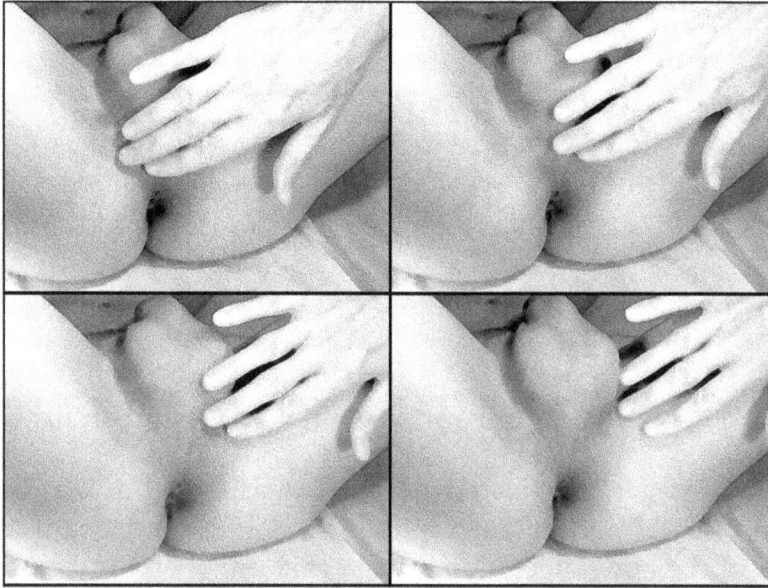

## VARIATIONS

☞ Perform the movement from left to right, and then from right to left.

☞ Change direction and stroke from front to back, starting from the scrotum going towards the anus, and vice versa.

# The Sewing Machine

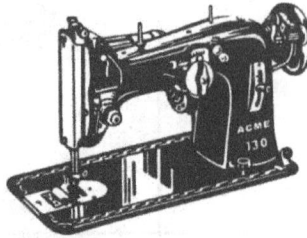

1. Position yourself in front of your partner, who is lying on his back.

2. Place your finger, lubricated or not, on the raphe just behind the scrotum. As we saw earlier, the raphe is the midline, or "seam" where the two halves of the body meet along the perineum.

3. Use your finger to quickly trace an imaginary line along this seam, as if you were trying to remove a stain with your finger. Apply a pressure between 2 and 5 on our scale.

4. After a second, repeat the same motion further along the raphe.

4. Repeat until your finger reaches his anus. Notice if his response changes as you move closer to his anus. If his body opens up more, it means he really likes it. If his body contracts and get tense, he either dislikes the sensation or might not be comfortable with playing so close to his anus.

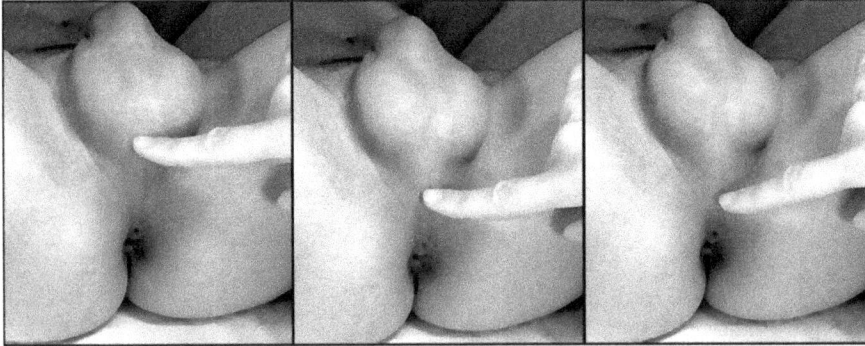

It's helpful to try different degrees of pressure when you perform this technique. Some men prefer gentle caresses while others like more firmness. It's usually more effective to begin gently and progressively increase pressure.

## VARIATIONS

☞ Move your finger along the raphe without lifting off.

☞ Start from the anus and move towards the scrotum.

☞ Caress the raphe from side to side, or zig-zig.

☞ Perform this technique and its variations using your tongue instead of your finger!

# Taking a Tissue

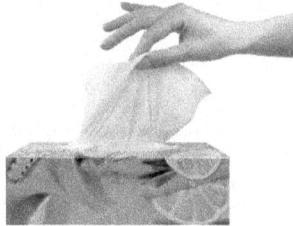

1. Place yourself near your partner so as to have access to his perineum. He can be standing or lying on his back.

2. Use your hand, lubricated or not, to caress his perineum using a motion similar to that you would use to retrieve a tissue from its box. When your fingers touch each other, your thumb should be on one side of the raphe, and your other fingers on the other side. Apply a pressure between 1 and 4 on our scale.

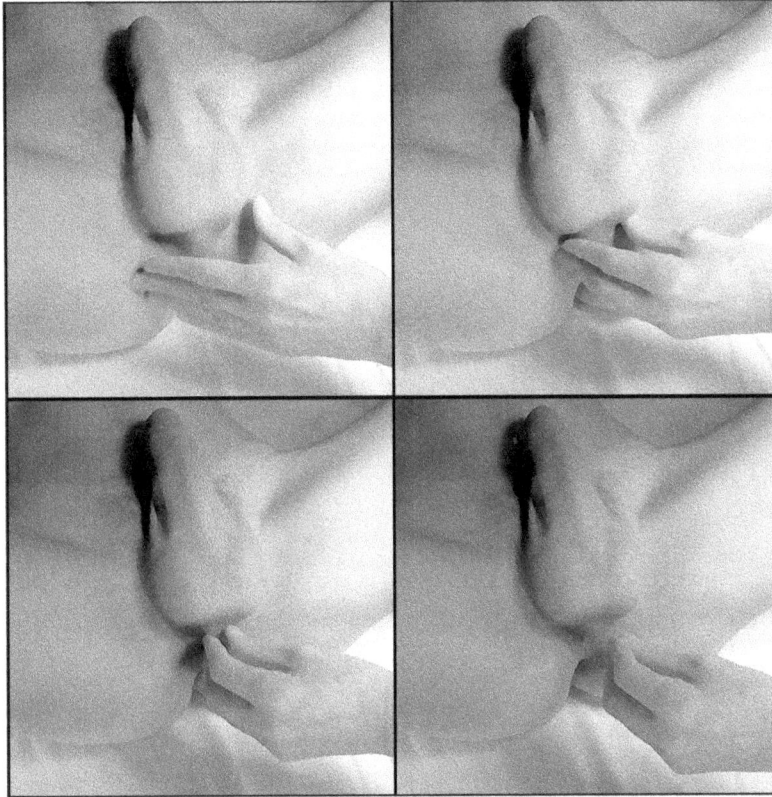

## VARIATION

☞ Perform this motion at different points along his perineum, and at different angles.

# The Aqua Park

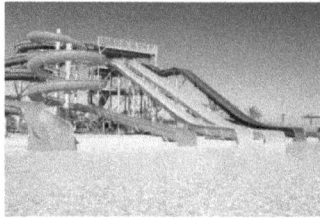

1. Stand in front of your partner, who is also standing, with his legs spread apart.

2. Slide your hand, lubricated or not, palm facing his perineum, between his legs until you are touching his buttocks. Use a pressure between 1 and 4 on our scale. Lubrication greatly amplifies the sensations!

3. Gently pull your hand back towards you.

4. Repeat steps 2 and 3. Your goal is always to maximize contact between your arm/hand and his perineum/buttocks.

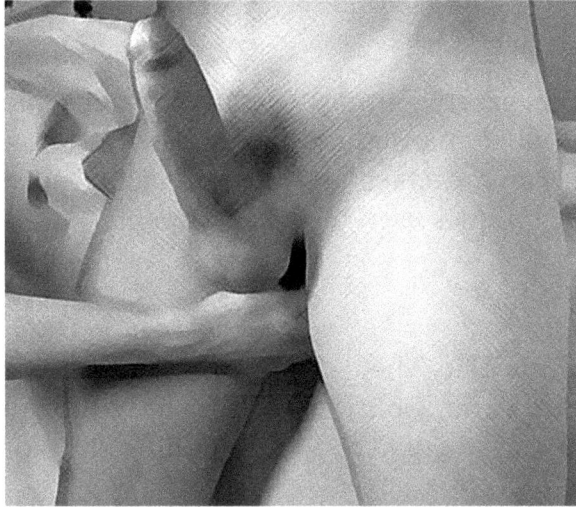

## VARIATIONS

☞ Rotate your wrist as you are sliding back and forth.

☞ Close your hand, making a fist, on some strokes.

☞ Do this from behind your partner instead of from the front.

☞ Stimulate his penis while doing the above.

💡 You can perform this technique in the shower, using a mild body wash gel or soap instead of lubricant. You'll both understand very soon where this technique gets its name!

# CARESSING THE PUBIS

Touching the pubis can greatly intensify your partner's pleasure. The following maneuvers do not produce particularly strong sensations when performed by themselves, but they can spectacularly heighten his sexual excitement when combined with other techniques used on his erect penis.

When caressing his erection:

☞ **Mmm!**: Simply place the palm of your hand on his pubis, applying a pressure between 1 and 4 on our scale. Gently move your hand away from the penis towards his navel, lightly pulling the skin over the pubis with it.

☞ **Raindrops**: Gently tap your fingers or your palm against his pubis.

☞ **Petting the tiger:** Stroke his pubis with your fingertips or your hand. Use your other hand to pull the erect penis to an angle away from the pubis, which allows you more room to work on his pubis and changes the sensations felt by his penis.

☞ **Sneaky Thumb:** When performing any technique where you are holding the base of the penis with one hand, use your thumb of that hand to gently press or stroke the pubis.

☞ **Little Kisses:** Kiss the pubis and adjacent areas.

☞ **Love It!**: Use your hands to slowly glide up your partner's thighs, stopping at and caressing his pubis with your fingers or palms.

# Between the Sheets

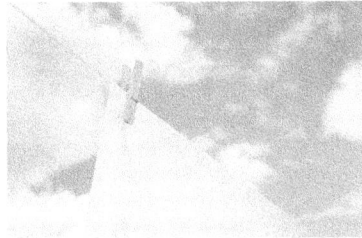

Most of the techniques presented so far can also be performed with the added help of a bed sheet. Placing a soft fabric between your hands and his erogenous zones can provide these delightful benefits:

- a softer experience for his penis, especially if your hands are rough

- a wider variety of pleasurable sensations

- allows greater fluidity in your movements

- permits you to skip using a lubricant

Underwear can produce the same effect, particularly lycra, microfiber and other ultra-soft fabrics.

This maneuver is better suited for preliminary caresses. As with all techniques, it can become monotonous if performed for too long.

# CARESSING THE ANUS
(...or Finding The Hidden Treasure Inside The Secret Cave)

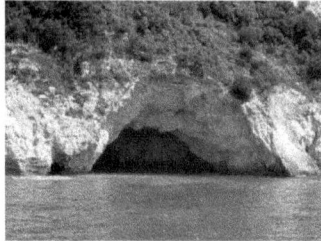

If you and your partner are open to exploring this road less-travelled, you'll discover ways to vastly intensify his pleasure. As this is a new and uncharted territory for many, we'll be introducing our techniques in the following order:

a) **exploratory techniques** (to see if he might like it)

b) **intermediate techniques** (because he's interested in going further)

c) **advanced techniques** (yeah, he likes it!)

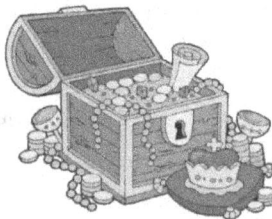

In this erogenous zone, as we've often seen before, it's usually preferable to do less than more. Proceeding too quickly can produce tense reactions or pain. We suggest you try out some of these techniques on yourself before trying them on your partner. This will give you a better idea of the sensitivity of the area (but don't expect to experience the same pleasure unless you are both sexually aroused and are a man with a prostate.)

For these caresses, it's important to take precautions with your fingernails, which can cause harm. If your partner enjoys caresses in the anal area, it's best to make sure the nail of the finger you will be using (usually the middle one) is well-trimmed and has no sharp edges. Don't forget to lubricate your finger well and repeatedly . . . it's essential!

## *Where to put your finger?*

Before inserting your finger into your partner's anus, it's essential to know where and how to place it. To ensure comfortable access to his sensual areas, you can start by having him lying down on his back. With the palm of your hand facing the ceiling, use your finger to very slowly and gently lubricate his anus and the adjacent areas. You should be able to feel his **external sphincter** muscles contract and relax as you massage the anus. The idea is to coax these muscles to relax as much as possible.

When the anus feels relaxed, apply more lubricant to your finger and very, very slowly insert your well-lubricated middle finger into his anus. As you do this, your finger may feel resistance as the external sphincter tightens up, in which case you should stop moving your finger until it relaxes again. If he experiences pain, try using more lubricant and proceed more slowly.

Once inside, your finger will be in a soft, warm canal, the **rectum**. As you slowly proceed, your finger might encounter another level of resistance from the **internal sphincter** muscles deeper inside the rectum. If this happens, stop moving and wait until it relaxes. You could also slowly pull your finger out and start again with more lubricant. This will allow the anus to get used to what you are doing. You can gently massage the external area around the anus to help the sphincters relax.

Once more than half your finger is inside, flex it (bend it slightly towards you) in order to follow the curve inside the rectum. The tip of your finger should be able to sense a firm mass above it on the other side of the membrane, slightly larger than the size of a cherry tomato half: this is the **prostate**. It's subtle and easy to miss! If your hands are small, your finger may be not long enough to feel it.

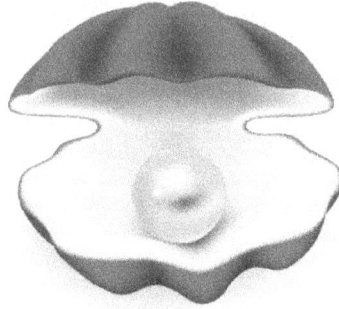

⚠️ The prostate is a very sensitive internal organ that is more vulnerable than skin and muscle. Its location inside the body normally provides protection from harmful impacts. Always treat it gently, never using more pressure than a 4 on our scale (squeezing a tube of toothpaste).

Many men prefer to have their erect penis stimulated (by themselves or their partner) while these techniques are performed on their anal erogenous zones. For these men, the anal techniques are not enjoyable without penis pleasure. Others may find anal stimulation alone to be abundantly pleasurable.

If your partner enjoys these types of caresses, slowly remove your finger from time to time. This will enhance his overall pleasure and allow his nerve endings to re-sensitize (and him to catch his breath!)

Before attempting the following techniques, we highly recommend you review the chapter on Exploring the Anal Erozone.

# Sit on my Knee!

**Exploratory technique - no penetration**

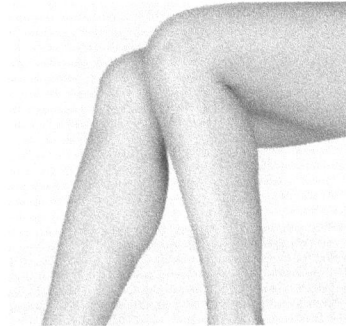

1. Sit on a chair or on the edge of a bed. Your knees should be bent at a 90° angle, and your feet firmly on the ground.

2. Ask your partner, who has an erection, to sit on one of your thighs, facing you.

3. Tell him he can stay seated on your thigh, or he can slightly raise and lower himself to increase and decrease the pressure of your thigh on his perineum and anus. He can also move or rub forwards and backwards along your thigh, or rock back and forth. What's happening? The pressure of his bodyweight on your thigh presses against his perineum and anus, and stimulates his prostate.

4. Use both hands to caress his penis and scrotum while he is exploring the above movements.

Don't be surprised if he starts rhythmically grinding his perineum and anus into your leg. If so, he's discovered the pleasure of prostate love! This is a good, wholesome introduction to the sensual rewards of prostate pleasure. And you may never look at sitting on someone's knee in the same way again!

# Around the Cavern Entrance

**Exploratory technique - no penetration**

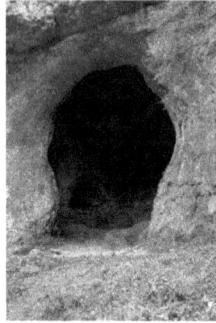

1. Position yourself to have comfortable access to your partner's anus while he has an erection.

2. Slowly and gently move your finger, lubricated or not, over the area surrounding his anus. This skin is richly innervated and very sensitive. As it is an area that has been taboo for many men, carefully observe his reactions to see whether or not you should continue with the next techniques.

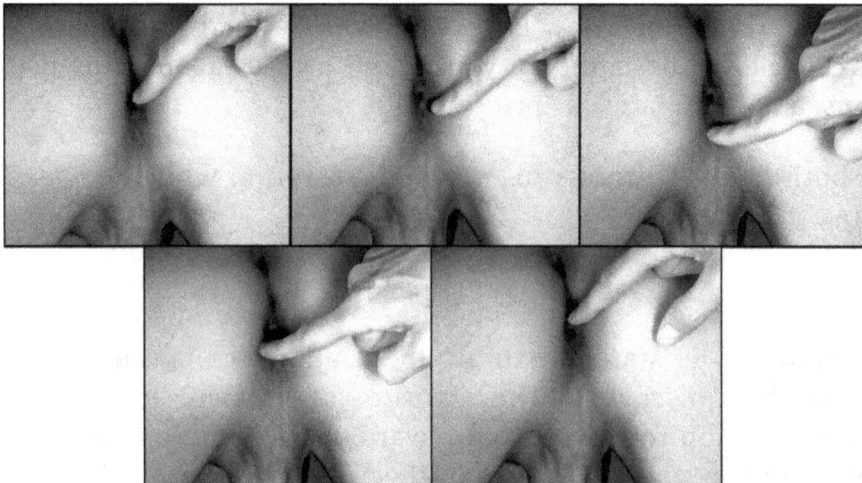

# The Doorbell

**Exploratory technique - no penetration**

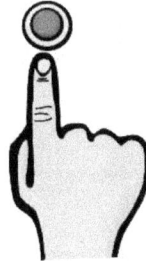

1. Delicately touch the anus with your index finger (lubrication is optional). Don't penetrate the anus, just loiter around the entrance outside. The presence of your finger is sufficiently stimulating. Be gentle.

2. At the same time, make sure his penis is being stimulated, either by his hand or your hand (or your mouth). Remove your finger for a couple of seconds every so often (this will make him want you to put it back!).

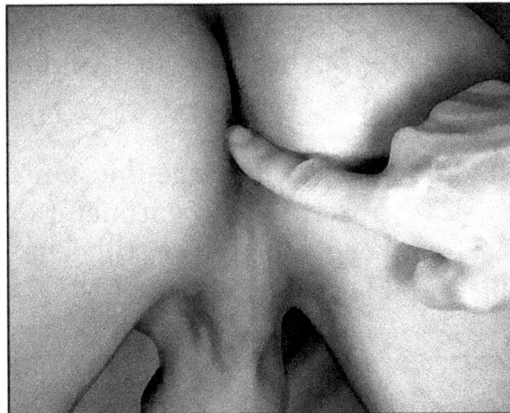

## *VARIATION*

☞ Gently vibrate your finger while touching the skin. Or slowly draw small circles.

# To Enter or Not To Enter?

**Exploratory technique - light penetration**

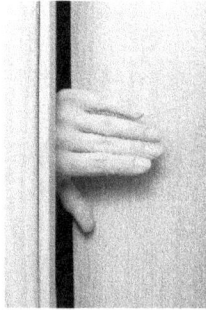

This technique is perfect for men who haven't had much experience with anal pleasure. It's gentle and only slightly intrusive. Watch your partner's reactions carefully and use this feedback to guide you.

1. Your partner can be lying on his back or standing up with his legs apart. Lubricate your middle finger well.

2. After using your middle finger to massage the skin around the anus for a minute, gently and slowly insert it one centimeter (a quarter inch) into your partner's anus. Then, keep your finger still. The simple presence of your finger creates pleasurable sensations.

3. After 10 or 15 seconds, slowly remove your finger.

## *VARIATION*

☞ When your fingertip is inside, move it a couple of millimeters (an eighth of an inch) to the right, and then to the left, or change the angle of your finger to get the same displacement.

# The Road Less Traveled

**Intermediate technique – with penetration**

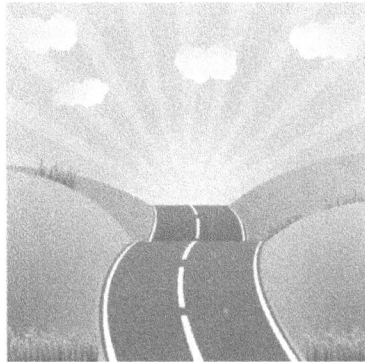

1. Lubricate your middle finger and his anus.

2. Position yourself to have comfortable access to your partner's anus. He is either lying on his back or standing with his legs apart.

3. Gently and slowly insert your lubricated finger until your second finger joint. Don't use pressure greater than 3 on our scale.

4. Gently wiggle your finger without moving the rest of your hand. Use the finger motion you would use when you want someone to "come here", except more slowly and with less flexion.

## *VARIATION*

☞ Once you have found the prostate, move your finger so that it taps it every couple of seconds.

# The Fingertip

**Intermediate technique – with penetration**

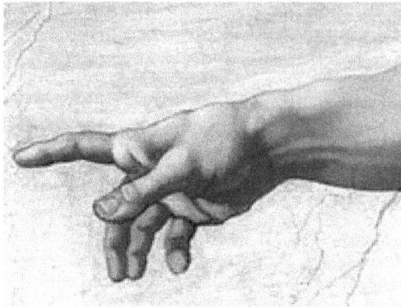

This technique is ideal for preparing your partner's anus for a deeper penetration.

1. Generously lubricate your index finger and his anus.

2. Gently touch your partner's anus with your index finger.

3. Slowly and gently slide your finger a few millimeters (a quarter inch) inside his anus. Keep it there for 5 seconds.

4. Slowly remove your finger.

5. Slowly insert it again, but go twice as far. Keep it there for 5 seconds.

6. Repeat the above, going a little further each time. The primary goal of this technique is not to go as deep as possible, but to gently stimulate the walls of the rectum. If he experiences pain, use more lubricant and perform the technique more slowly.

Try this on yourself! You'll gain a better idea of the sensations your partner will feel.

When beginning this technique, never insert or remove your finger quickly as this can be painful. Moderate your movements until you are both comfortable with this technique, or you may never get another invitation! And that would be a shame because great sexual power can be wielded by those who have mastered these techniques!

# The Serpent

**Advanced technique – with penetration**

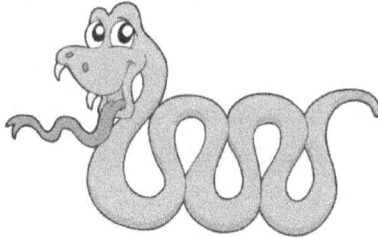

This technique involves making meandering, serpentine movements with your middle finger.

1. Position yourself in front of your partner who is lying on his back or standing with legs apart.

2. Generously lubricate your middle finger and his anus.

3. With your palm facing you, slowly and gently insert your middle finger completely into your partner's anus.

4. Using a pressure of no more than 3 on our scale, move your fingertip back and forth as you slowly pull your finger out, tracing a meandering path that a snake uses when it moves. At some point it will trace over the prostate.

5. Stop when the first joint of your finger arrives at the anal opening.

6. Insert it completely again, repeating the above movements.

## VARIATIONS

☞ While performing the above movements, use your other hand to massage and caress his perineum.

☞ Instead of tracing the path of a serpent, use your finger to write words, and even write out your name! Make it a romantic moment to cherish forever!

# The Metronome

**Advanced technique – with penetration**

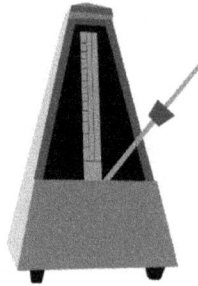

In this technique, you'll be reproducing the movement of the pendulum in a metronome.

1. Lubricate your middle finger and his anus generously.

2. Position yourself in front of your partner, who is either lying on his back or standing.

3. With your palm facing you, slowly insert your finger into his rectum all the way, or as far as he is comfortable.

4. Gently move your finger back and forth as if it was the pendulum of a metronome. It should take at least 2 seconds to swing each way.

## *VARIATION*

☞ At step 4, trace circles with your finger around and over the prostate instead of sweeping it back and forth. If your finger performs this movement during ejaculation, you'll feel the contractions of his prostate.

# Side Order

**Advanced technique – with penetration**

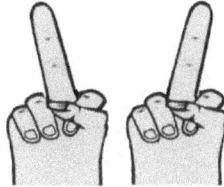

1. Lubricate your middle finger and his anus generously.

2. Position yourself in front of your partner, who is either lying on his back or standing.

3. With your palm facing you, slowly insert your finger into his rectum all the way, or as far as he is comfortable.

4. Move your finger to one side of the rectum. Apply a pressure between 1 and 3 on our scale.

5. Gently explore this area, sliding your fingertip along the canal. Only your finger moves, not your hand.

6. Do the same on the other side.

# In and Out

**Advanced technique – with penetration**

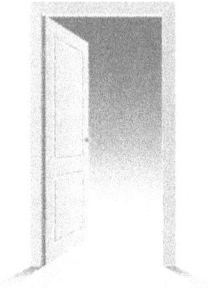

This technique involves inserting and withdrawing your middle finger from your partner's anus, and requires deliberate gentleness (unless you are directed otherwise!).

1. Lubricate your middle finger generously, as well as your partner's anus.

2. Position yourself in front of your partner, who is either lying on his back or standing.

3. With your palm facing you, slowly insert your finger into his rectum all the way. We suggest you take up to 20 seconds for the first penetration. Going faster may cause his sphincters to tighten up. Do not exceed a pressure of 3 on our scale.

4. When it is in all the way, wait a few seconds, then slowly withdraw your finger. Repeat as desired.

Take your time! For many, speed is inversely proportional to pleasure! For others, rapid finger thrusts are the ticket to nirvana.

## VARIATIONS

☞ Do not withdraw completely. Leave your fingertip inside his anus.

☞ When your finger is in all the way, massage his prostate a few seconds if you're able.

☞ Some men may enjoy two fingers at once. More than that, a dildo comes in handy.

## The Zen of Dawdling in the Doorway

*The following vignette describes a Zen-like state of mind that you might find helpful when caressing your partner's anus.*

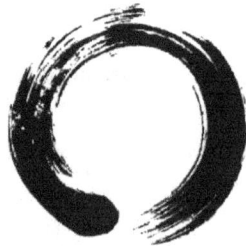

His penis is erect. You're stroking it slowly.

You slide your other hand under his balls, caressing them. You brush them with your wrist as your hand slowly glides further back between his legs. Your fingers caress his perineum, weaving back and forth across his raphe, that line that separates his body halves. Your fingertips tease the skin as they gently and slowly edge towards the anus, following the raised ridge along the Axis of Pleasure. Your index finger arrives at the anus and stops there for a few seconds. For you, it's not much, but for him, you're at the doorway to a place far more private than his penis, so there needs to be a little period of adjustment. Be patient.

After waiting ten, twenty, thirty seconds, gently move your finger. Not inside, but outside. Apply a little pressure at the doorway, like a cat's paw.

All the while, you're still stroking his penis, or he is.

Your finger grazes the entrance of the anus. Let it move towards the center of the hole, then back away. No rush. Your finger teases, it loiters. It touches, it doesn't touch. You run your finger along the raphe again. Then back to the hole, intimating it may go inside, but not doing so.

You wiggle your finger on the anal opening. If you're using lubricant and you don't have sharp nails, your finger can almost slide in. Watch his reaction.

You see he likes it, you tease again a few times. Then, your finger "accidentally" slips inside a bit, then comes back out.

Your finger progressively slides inside a little further each time, until a few minutes later, your whole finger is inside. You feel his prostate and slowly swirl your finger around it.

He is now in an altered state.

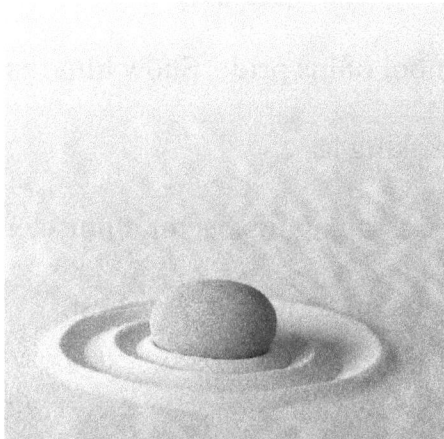

# Haiku

*Slow probing finger*

*moving towards his center*

*deep total pleasure*

# CARESSING OTHER EROGENOUS ZONES

## Chest

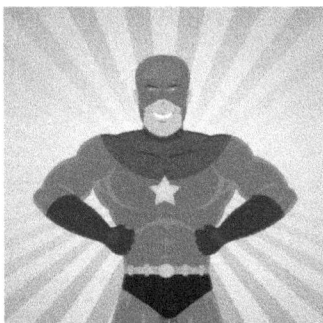

A man's chest is often a symbol of his pride. Show him that you like his chest by:

☞ Rubbing and stroking it.

☞ Squeezing and massaging his pectoral muscles.

☞ Sliding your hands up and down his chest.

## Nipples

Have you ever asked the question: Why do men have nipples?

There are 2 answers. You can pick the one you prefer:

**Answer 1:** Females need them to suckle their young, and nipples develop in the fetus before hormones differentiate the baby's sex. So they are already there before male physical characteristics develop.

**Answer 2:** Because it's fun when they're played with.

Nipples, as many men will attest, are an important erogenous zone. Many men like to have them touched, licked, flicked, pulled, pinched, bitten or even pierced. Some prefer it gentle, others like it rough. Like women, men have an areola, the outer circle of sensitive tissue, and a nipple at the center. There are some men who do not experience pleasure from stimulation of their nipples.

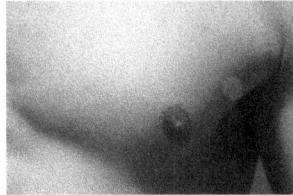

Find out if your man likes these techniques, and how much pressure to use:

☞ **Rubbing:** Start by gently brushing the nipples with your finger. Rub up and down, or in circles.

☞ **Flicking:** Gently flick his nipple with your finger. Start gently as he may not like this.

☞ **Pinching**: Squeeze his areola or his nipple between your fingers, using a pressure from 1 to 6 on our scale.

☞ **Pulling:** You can pull his areola or his nipple away from his body, or in different directions. Use a pressure from 1 to 6 on our scale.

☞ **Licking:** Sometimes your hands are just too busy doing other pleasurable things to him, so you have to use your mouth! Very sensual.

☞ **Biting:** Light and irregular pressure using your teeth can be exciting, especially while his penis is being stimulated. Just make sure you don't draw blood!

## Stomach

Many men can become aroused by having their stomach rubbed. In addition to being very soothing, it can help relax the diaphragm and the abdominal muscles, allowing him to be more "in the moment". This can also stimulate the pubis, the erogenous zone we explored earlier.

## Neck

Do you like having your neck kissed? Or having someone's face muzzling the side of your neck? As we all know, the neck has very sensitive nerve endings, and some find neck contact very arousing. Be careful, it can be ticklish!

☞ Caressing or kissing his neck can create a mind-blowing experience when combined with other techniques.

# Multi-zone Techniques

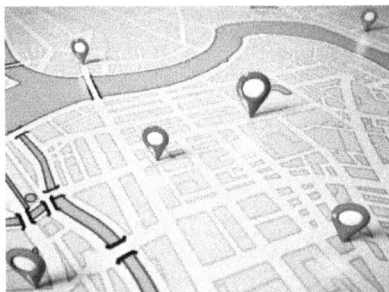

You should be ready now to discover a set of techniques that involve caressing multiple erogenous zones at once.

These techniques are particularly rewarding because you can use them to send overwhelming jolts of pleasure throughout your partner's nervous system. With the right touch, the simultaneous stimulation of multiple pleasurable nerve endings will blow his mind like never before. Be prepared for a wild reaction!

Some of the techniques may require greater dexterity, as they require the use of both your hands and sometimes another part of your body. In this guide, we've focused almost completely on the use of your hands to stimulate your partner's body. However, since most readers have only two hands, you'll need to use other body parts for these techniques. One body part that comes in handy (please forgive the pun!) is your mouth, which can be used as a substitute for a hand in many of the techniques we've covered so far.

We recommend you start with some of the preceding single-zone techniques before attempting these multi-zone ones. And you may need to practice a few times before mastering them (he probably won't mind!).

# The Prisoner

- **PERINEUM**
- **PENIS**
- **ANAL EROZONE**

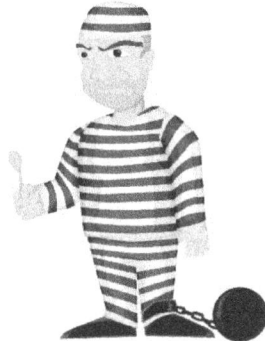

1. Stand behind your partner, who is also standing.

2. Ask him to start playing with his penis.

3. While he is masturbating, slide your hand (lubricated or not), between his legs, taking care to caress the crack of his buttocks with your fingers.

4. Slowly, keep gliding your hand forward. Your wrist should now be in contact with his Anal Erozone. (Don't be shy -- he's enjoying it.) Aim for maximum contact between your hand, wrist and forearm with his body. You can also slowly rotate your hand and forearm as you glide, further stimulating his Axis of Pleasure along its length.

5. Keep gliding your fingers forward along his perineum and eventually they will touch his scrotum. Caress the raphe with your fingers as they move forward. Then, cup his scrotum with your hand and caress it.

6. Still slowly moving forward in a smooth, uninterrupted glide, your fingers will reach the base of his penis. He may stop masturbating at this point (too much pleasure!) You can now caress his penis with the same hand, or with your other hand.

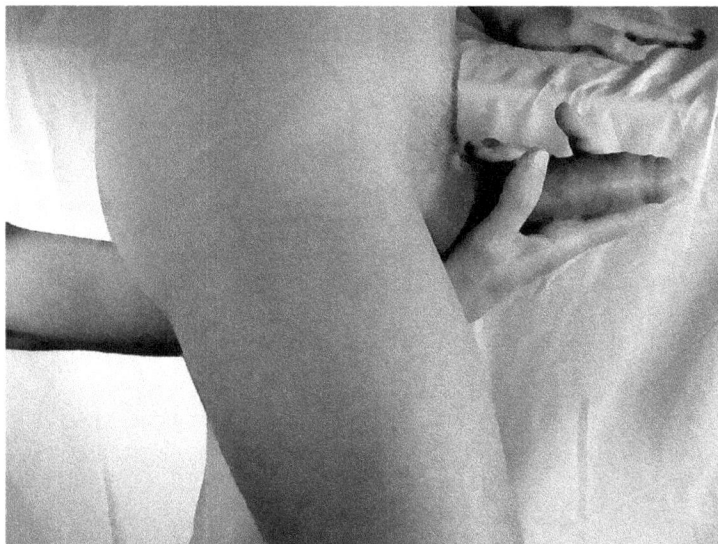

7. Once your hand reaches the tip of his penis, gently masturbate it. After a few seconds, reverse direction and repeat the same movements as you slowly withdraw your hand. Try to maintain as much contact as possible between your body parts and his. You can exert a pressure between 1 and 4 on our scale to his perineum with your forearm.

8. Repeat back and forth as desired.

## VARIATION

☞ You can also perform this technique from behind your partner when he is kneeling on the bed.

💡 If you want to add another level of excitement, you can handcuff or tie your partner's hands together (hence the reason for this technique's name). If you secure his hands behind his back, he won't be able to masturbate... but maybe that's what the prison warden wants!

# Scaling the Inner Thighs

- **PERINEUM**
- **LEGS**
- **INTERNAL CREASE OF THE THIGHS**

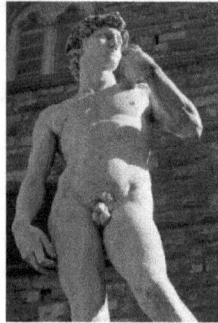

1. Your partner can be lying on his back or standing.

2. Place one or more fingers of one hand on the inner thigh of your partner, near his knee.

3. Slowly move your hand towards the internal crease of his thigh.

4. Continue this movement, and gently caress his perineum with your fingertips.

5. Keep moving towards his other inner thigh and glide your hand along his thigh down to the knee.

6. Repeat the above steps in reverse.

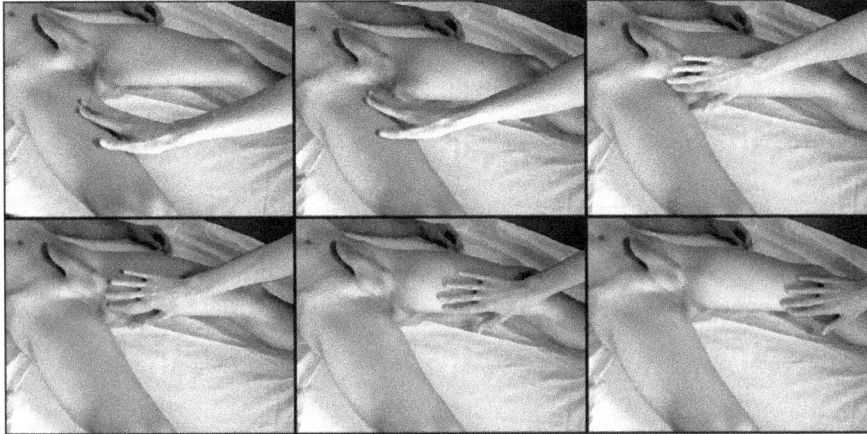

## VARIATIONS

☞ Instead of your fingertips, use the palm of your hand or your tongue.

☞ Once your fingers reach his perineum, take the opportunity to perform one of the perineum techniques described earlier.

👓 *You can use a lubricant but this requires the inner thighs to be lubricated as well. This is a great technique during a massage!*

# The Diamond

- PERINEUM
- PENIS
- SCROTUM
- PUBIS

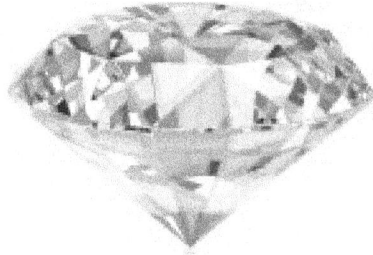

This technique allows you to caress the perineum, pubis, scrotum and penis all at once. Not bad for such a simple but elegant technique!

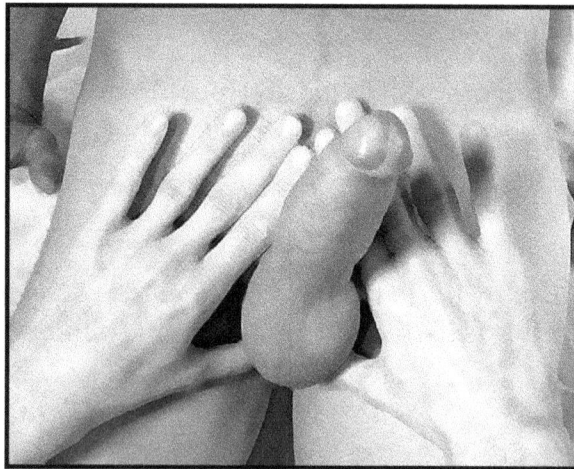

1. Lubricate your hands if desired.

2. Place your thumbs on his perineum near the scrotum. His scrotum may hang down atop your thumbs, which are lightly touching each other.

3. Place the tips of your index fingers on his pubis, with the tips touching each other. Your thumbs and index fingers should form a diamond shape.

4. Caress his perineum or his scrotum with your thumbs.

5. At the same time, caress his pubis with your index fingers.

6. Stimulate his penis while doing the above in one or more of these ways:

☞ Using your mouth.

☞ He masturbates.

☞ Perform a **Half-diamond**. This is like a diamond but using only one hand. Use your free hand to stimulate his penis using one of the techniques we've already described.

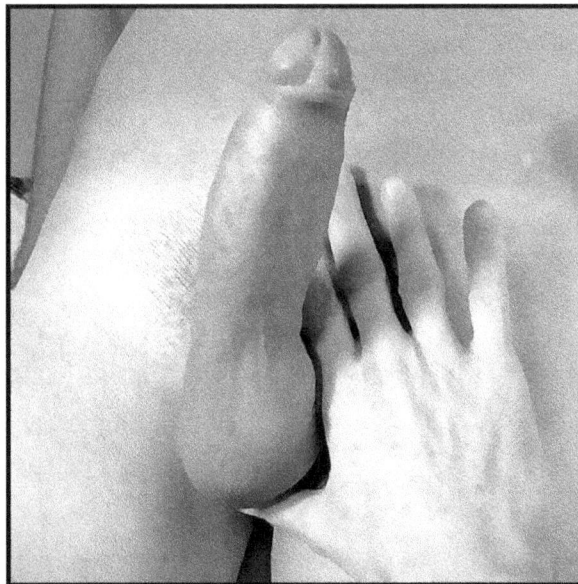

☞ From time to time, remove your hand from the Diamond to caress the penis for a few strokes.

# The J

- **PERINEUM**
- **SCROTUM**
- **PENIS**

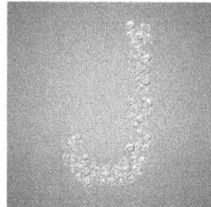

1. Stand in front of your partner, who is also standing, with his legs apart.

2. Slide your hand, lubricated or not, between his legs, with your fingers and the palm of your hand caressing his perineum.

3. Your palm should exert a pressure on his perineum between 1 and 5 on our scale.

4. At the same time, position your wrist so that it applies a gentle pressure on the front side of the base of his penis. Make sure you don't squeeze his testicles.

5. Rub the front of his penis with your forearm.

6. With your other hand, you can:

- apply gentle pressure on his Leverage Point.

- perform other techniques on his penis.

- send a text message.

# The Hook

- **PERINEUM**
- **ANUS**
- **RECTUM**

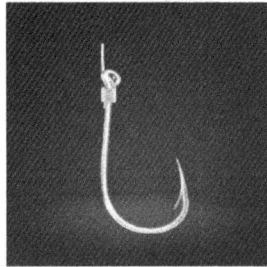

1. Position yourself in front of your partner, who is also standing, with his legs apart.

2. Slide your hand between his legs at the groin.

3. Place your index finger, lubricated or not, on and around the outside of his anus and caress that area.

4. With the palm of the same hand, apply light pressure on his perineum.

## *VARIATIONS*

☞ You can gently move your palm around, caressing his perineum, while keeping your index finger on and around his anus.

☞ Shake your hand like a vibrator while performing this technique.

☞ If your partner is open to the idea, you can insert your lubricated finger inside his rectum.

# The Carrousel

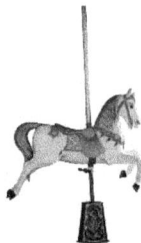

1. Place yourself in front of your partner, who is standing, kneeling on the bed, or lying on his side.

2. Stretch out your hand, wrist and forearm, lubricated or not, in a straight line.

3. Slide your hand between his legs along his groin. The side of your hand, wrist and forearm should slide along his perineum, using a pressure between 1 and 4 on our scale.

4. While caressing his perineum, begin to change the angle of your wrist so that your hand caresses his Anal Erozone. You can use a stronger pressure, up to a 6 on our scale, on the external Anal Erozone as long as it is generally diffused over a larger area (by using the side of your hand as compared to a finger, which could be uncomfortable). If he is standing, you can apply even more pressure with your hand, so that you are supporting some of his weight, if you are able to.

5. With your other hand, stimulate his penis using one of his preferred techniques or suggest that he masturbate or caress himself.

6. Massage his Anal Erozone with the side of your hand, using one of these movements:

- small circular movements.

- applying pressure in intervals (3 seconds on, 3 seconds off).

• back and forth movements.

• rotate your forearm along its Axis so that different parts of it caress his perineum and his Anal Erozone.

In addition to producing cascades of pleasure in the sensitive nerve endings of his scrotum, perineum and Anal Erozone, this technique also stimulates his hidden penis and, indirectly, his prostate.

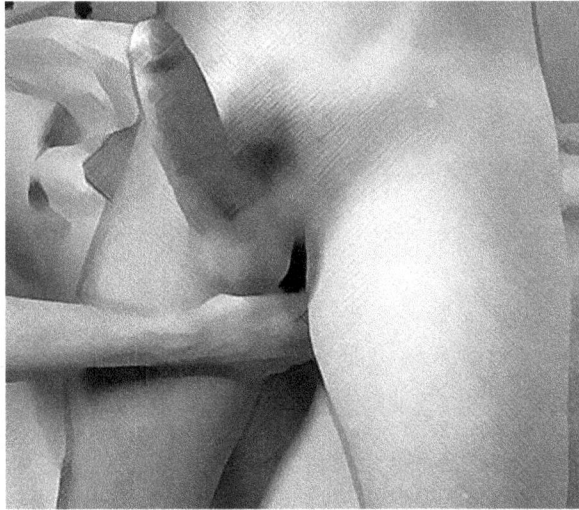

## VARIATION

☞ While your forearm and wrist are caressing his Axis of Pleasure, grip and squeeze his buttock with your hand. It's a wonderful feeling for him.

This technique can be performed with or without lubricant. Try it both ways, as each brings about very different sensations.

# Trifecta!

- **PERINEUM**
- **PENIS**
- **ANAL EROZONE**
- **PROSTATE**

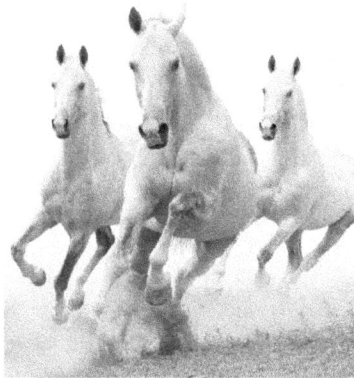

Once you've mastered the previous techniques, you can try this one, which combines three at once:

1. Begin by performing oral sex.

2. At the same time, slowly insert a lubricated finger into his anus and massage his prostate. You can use a finger condom on the penetrating finger, if desired.

3. With your other hand, caress his scrotum and perineum.

## *VARIATION*

☞ At step 3, instead of caressing his scrotum and perineum with your other hand, use it to encircle the base of his penis. Stroke the penis up and down, or in a gentle corkscrew motion.

☝ If you don't want him to come in your mouth, tell him before you start, as this technique can trigger orgasm very quickly.

⚠ For hygienic reasons, make sure you don't touch anything with the finger you inserted into his anus. If either of you gets tired of the anal penetration, either remove the condom from your finger, or wash your hands.

# Where to Start?

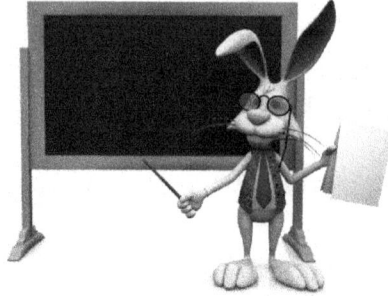

You now have the knowledge required to transport your partner to unparalleled heights of ecstasy using only your hands. If you have not yet begun to put this knowledge into practice, now is the time! Some readers may feel a bit of information overload or anxiety over remembering the many erogenous zones and how to best stimulate each. If so, start by choosing one or two techniques that you'd like to try out with your partner. As with learning any new skill, it's best to take your time and go at your own pace.

To master the techniques and gain confidence, you could alternatively start by practicing on a dildo or object that resembles a penis. This will allow you to mentally integrate the steps of each technique, much like a pianist who rehearses a piece before performing it on stage.

Then, gradually add other techniques to your lovemaking. Don't expect to master everything the first time. It's quite likely you'll need to review the steps of some techniques more than once. All art involving skill takes time and practice!

In the event that you've learned to perform the techniques on the same man, and then find yourself with a new partner, you will likely need to return to basics and reassess how your new partner responds to the various factors that make up a technique, such as pressure, timing, etc. As we have already mentioned, every man is different!

# Perfect your Artistry

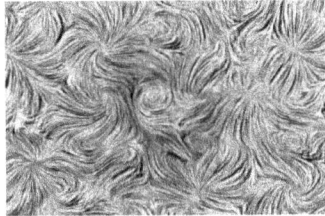

If you follow what has been presented in this book to the letter, you'll possess exceptional skills in the art of erotic touch.

We do, however, encourage you to refine your newly developed skills to an even higher level, bringing out the artist in you.

A budding painter must first learn basic painting techniques in order to experiment with them. Once the painter has mastered them, he or she can apply them at will. The goal is no longer to master the techniques but to transcend them and express oneself in one's own unique way. This is when the painter truly becomes an artist.

Similarly, you'll likely begin by discovering and experimenting with the various techniques in this book. Your first goal might be to master them in order to increase the pleasure of your partner. The ultimate goal, however, is to reach a point where you can express what you feel for your partner through your hands in an inspired and creative way. You'll both find yourselves benefiting from more authentic communication, deeper intimacy and a stronger connection.

# Important Message for the Whole World

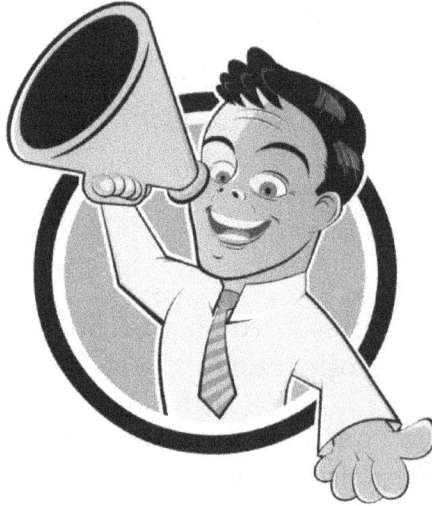

There is a great danger that threatens to ruin the pleasure that so many of us are striving to provide, and we genuinely believe it's in the public interest to mention it here: be careful of the harm that can be wrought by . . . your teeth! Although this book focuses on caresses made with your hands, you may find yourself sometimes performing oral sex on your partner. One needs to be ever mindful to avoid contact between your teeth and his penis. This occurs far more often than we think, even if you firmly believe it's not true in your case. The best thing to do is to ask your partner if he feels your teeth. By addressing this unspoken and much-neglected peril in a thoughtful and vigilant manner, we, together, can make ours a better world!

# Adventure Awaits!

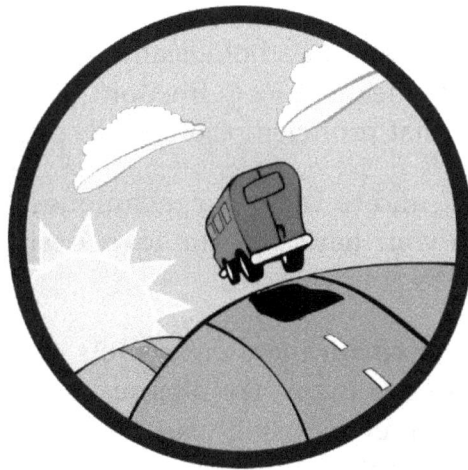

You've now acquired invaluable knowledge about male erogenous zones and if you've practiced what you've learned, you should also have developed some impressive erotic skills. We hope you've been encouraged by your partner's responses to your erotic touch and that you'll continue to practice and build on your expertise.

You can combine the many techniques we've presented to form an infinite number of possible combinations. However, if there is any domain where one should not be struggling to accomplish something, but rather just be having fun, this is it. So please don't take it all too seriously...the important thing is to have fun and trust your instincts.

If, throughout your experimenting, you've regularly sought feedback from your partner (in words, moans or on a scale of 1 to 10), you should by now have established more direct and open communication with him, developed greater intimacy and gained a deeper understanding of what pleases him. This process will hopefully allow you to express your own sexual needs and wishes more clearly and openly as well. As we said earlier, the general principles of giving pleasure with erotic touch are equally applicable to you. Setting an example of how to touch and give pleasure often leads to bountiful reciprocation.

The benefits extend well beyond sexual pleasure. A healthy sex life is important for overall health, both physically and psychologically. Having more options in how to engage in sexual relations means more freedom for you, in addition to the confidence and satisfaction that proficient erotic skills provide.

We invite you to be creative and to vary your techniques. Why not invent your own techniques to express with your hands all the love, desire and respect you feel for the partner who surrenders to your caresses!

We're very happy to have shared with you our secrets of erotic touch. We hope that our playful approach inspires you to take all the time you need to practice this sensual pursuit and that you'll enjoy using your new abilities to build and multiply your partner's pleasure to unrivalled climaxes.

Your ultimate success will be to find yourself with a smiling, satisfied partner, ready to do anything to make you happy, because he knows that he's in excellent hands!

Notes

www.ingramcontent.com/pod-product-compliance
Lightning Source LLC
Chambersburg PA
CBHW081413270326
41931CB00015B/3260